« THE DOUBLE BIND OF DISABILITY »

The Double Bind of Disability

How Medical Technology Shapes Bodily Authority

REBECCA MONTELEONE

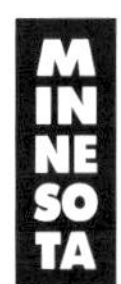

University of Minnesota Press
Minneapolis
London

Published by the University of Minnesota Press
111 Third Avenue South, Suite 290
Minneapolis, MN 55401-2520
http://www.upress.umn.edu

ISBN 978-1-5179-1767-8 (hc)
ISBN 978-1-5179-1768-5 (pb)

A Cataloging-in-Publication record for this book is available from the Library of Congress.

Printed in the United States of America on acid-free paper

UMP BmB 2025

Contents

Abbreviations

AANS	American Association of Neurological Surgeons
APS	artificial pancreas system
cfDNA	cell-free DNA
CGM	continuous glucose monitor
DBS	deep brain stimulation
DIYAPS	do-it-yourself artificial pancreas system
FDA	U.S. Food and Drug Administration
IPG	internal pulse generator
ISF	insulin sensitivity factor
MDI	multiple daily injections
NIPS	noninvasive prenatal screening
PGT	prenatal genetic screening and testing
T1D	type 1 diabetes

Introduction

Caught in the Double Bind

Abby

Abby is thirty-three years old and pregnant. She has spent the past several years navigating fertility treatments. Throughout the process of conceiving and carrying this pregnancy, Abby and her husband have resisted genetic testing to learn about their likelihood of bearing a child with a congenital difference such as Down syndrome. They cite their Catholic faith and their strong desire for a child as reason enough to avoid it, explicitly associating testing with pregnancy termination. Abby tells me, "We're not doing [genetic testing] because we're good Catholics, and because we love this baby, and because it doesn't matter and it's not going to change anything, and we have to look like we're good people who don't care and are going to love our baby."

However, as Abby has visited online pregnancy forums, done research on her own, and witnessed many discussions on genetic testing, she began to feel a different pressure: the pressure to prove herself as a responsible mother, despite many conflicting messages about what that means. She tells me about other prospective parents in the pregnancy forums:

> People [are] saying, "Well, it doesn't matter." I'm like, "You're right. It doesn't matter to me, either. And now I have to prove that. I have to prove that I'm going to love my baby no matter what and not do this testing." But then the other people are saying, "No, you have to prove that you want to be prepared for your baby and do everything you can before they get here." And [I'm] like, "Oh yeah, I have to prove that I'm going to be the best mom and do everything I can." So, it's about proving how much

> you love your baby and that it's just as much or more than the person next to you.

Despite all of the time and thought Abby and her husband had put into preparing for this decision, she was still caught unaware when the moment came. At the beginning of an appointment with her obstetrician, a medical assistant who was drawing her blood asked offhandedly if she'd like another vial taken for noninvasive prenatal screening. Abby recalls being flustered, her husband still out parking the car:

> It was just so nonchalant. They did my weight, and they did my blood pressure, and they took my blood, and then I went back for the ultrasound. We weren't meeting about it or anything, it was just, "Do you want me to take this extra tube of blood? Yes, or no?" And that was the whole conversation about it. . . . I wasn't prepared for it . . . I would've come in with all my questions, all my papers or whatever. But in the moment, I was just like, deer in headlights, like, "Okay, sure."

Mary

Mary and I sit in the public library, chatting about brain implants. She is an author living in the Southwest, writing about her experiences with early-onset Parkinson's disease. In 2012, she underwent surgery for deep brain stimulation, in which electrodes were implanted that now send electrical impulses to the areas of her brain that control gait, balance, and tremor. During our two and a half hours together, Mary shares both the joys and the frustrations of her device. While she is pleased with the implant overall, she also expresses disbelief at how disconnected the designers of these devices and the clinicians who oversee their use are from the disabled people who use them. For example, her implant is powered by a battery pack that rests just under her clavicle. Because the battery pack has a square edge, when she raises her arm, it juts out. "They don't think about how you're going to shave your underarm," she laughs.

She and her husband, Barry, who joins us for the conversation, lament that there are so few opportunities for people with Parkinson's to share their knowledge with clinicians and designers. Mary tells me:

> When you go to a conference you've got five hundred people with Parkinson's, and you got two experts up there on the stage with their PowerPoint going "blah blah blah blah." I've often said if you could get five hundred medical professionals and force them to sit and listen to twenty Parkinson's patients up there on the stage, the amount of info they would learn would be amazing.

Barry quickly follows up with, "Except none of them would come."

Near the end of our conversation, Mary shares her thoughts on a new device in development. It is an updated version of a patient remote, a controller that allows the user to adjust the level of stimulation from an implant within certain parameters. Where previous models have used analog buttons, this new design features a sleek touch screen. Mary rolls her eyes. For many people with Parkinson's, tremors and fine motor dexterity issues mean that touch screens are difficult, if not impossible, to use. The irony is palpable: The sole function of this piece of technology is to enable user control over a medical device, and it is unusable by its intended audience. Barry says, "If they had talked to the patient first, they would've pointed that out right away. You're going in the wrong direction here. People with Parkinson's should be the ones who are designing these things."

Carolyn

Carolyn has seen doctors and medical technology companies make a lot of promises in the fifty-five years since she was diagnosed with type 1 diabetes (T1D). She remembers her doctor telling her, half a century ago, that a cure was only two years away. "And I started to kind of give up on that after about ten years," she tells me. "I thought, 'Well, [my doctor] is lying.'" In the intervening years, Carolyn has not waited for a cure. Instead, she began a blog, wrote a book, and started a support group out of her living room. She often discusses the exhaustion and isolation of monitoring and managing food, exercise, blood sugar, and insulin. "There's really very few, if any, other diseases that are this user-intensive and complicated," she says. "And no matter what you do, you're not going to get the same results. So, it's terribly frustrating." On top of those internal frustrations, she adds, is the lack of empathy and investment that many with T1D face in clinical settings, especially when their health care professionals have no personal lived experience with diabetes. "They are blamed," she tells me of people with T1D who struggle to control it. "They're just burned out. They're tired. They're overwhelmed by it." She finds echoes of this apathy in the companies that develop diabetes technology, saying, "In terms of being patient-centric, they're just not . . . they're businesses. They go home at five and the rest of us still are managing diabetes."

She contrasts this blame and lack of understanding with the support she has found in community with people creating and using do-it-yourself artificial pancreas systems. Using a continuous glucose monitor, an insulin pump, and a smart device to run an open-source algorithm, these homemade systems automate insulin delivery based on input data, relieving users of much of the day-to-day cognitive burden of T1D. In addition to the change such a system has made to her quality of life, Carolyn celebrates the community itself, telling me, "I'm hooked to this community. And I am so beyond grateful for what people do in it. I don't even know how to describe how amazing it is." In direct contrast to being told by clinicians to wait for a cure while simultaneously bearing the brunt of responsibility for staying alive, she says, "the blessing of the do-it-yourself community is it's impatient. . . . It's like, 'Okay, don't tell us to wait.'"

The Tangled Knowledge Politics of Medical Technology

On the surface, Abby, Mary, and Carolyn have little in common. They do not come from similar geographic locations or socioeconomic backgrounds. Their ages range across thirty-odd years. They have vastly different reasons for using medical technology, and the technologies they use vary in their mechanisms, their invasiveness, and how long the user is in contact with them.[1] It may seem that little can be learned from putting these anecdotes in conversation that would not be learned from examining each alone. I argue, however, that these stories taken together expose new relationships among disability, authority, knowledge, and responsibility. Most importantly, they reveal the role that medical technology plays in producing these meanings. The stories shared by Abby, Mary, and Carolyn—using prenatal genetic screening, deep brain stimulation, and do-it-yourself artificial pancreas systems, respectively—typify the strained, complex, and evolving knowledge politics produced by and mediated through medical technology.

Drawing deeply from disability studies, feminist science and technology studies, and medical sociology, I present here an interdisciplinary exploration of accountability, authority, and ability through close qualitative examinations of these three technologies. I argue that in a society that increasingly values the professional medical class and technologists as adjudicators of acceptable embodiment, how individuals experience themselves—their bodies, their minds, their relationships—is dismissed or called into question when it comes into conflict with medical authority. Disabled people are expected to defer to expert authority while also being held responsible for managing and adapting their bodyminds to pass in a world built by and for nondisabled people.[2] Both this deference and this accountability deny embodied and experiential knowledge. As medicine defines the parameters of ability, so too does it define and animate the obligation to approximate the nondisabled, productive bodymind. Medical technologies, from preventive screening to advanced prosthetics, have come to play a key role in the articulation and enactment of ability and disability. Ultimately, as I will show, these technologies perpetuate epistemic invalidation and ableism while simultaneously displacing ableism's pressures for individual users. Within these restrictive sociotechnical systems, medical technology users are imagining new social, political, and material arrangements, ones that resist neoliberal individualization, redefine boundaries of control and acceptable bodyminds, and explicitly embrace experiential and embodied knowledge.

In recent years, the rhetoric of individual autonomy, independence, and consumer choice has come to animate the design and use of many medical technologies. With this discourse of increased autonomy comes an accompanying discourse of personal responsibility. Essentially, for disabled people (or the prospective parents of disabled people), the promise of technologically enabled independence comes packaged with the obligation to pursue it. Importantly, configuring disability as detectable, manageable, and curable through medical technology undermines constructions of disability as a social, political, and collective phenomenon.

Therefore, the implications of medical technologies extend far beyond the clinic. Previous research has found that the subordination of embodied and experiential expertise and the insistence on personal responsibility result in harmful design, insufficient clinical care, misdiagnosis and mistreatment, guilt, and abuse.[3] Taking these findings for granted, I seek to answer two interlinked questions: (1) How do medical technologies mediate the meaning of disability and experiences of nonnormativity? (2) How do knowledge and responsibility get constructed and enacted in the interaction between disabled and nonnormative bodyminds and medical technologies?

The technologies I analyze in this book are connected through data, knowledge, and choice. Since the mid-twentieth century, laboratory medicine—which relies on biological detection and bodily quantification rather than clinical observation and judgment—has become central in Western medical practice.[4] Alongside this material transformation, new moral regimes emerged, demanding that individuals collect as many data as possible about their bodyminds in pursuit of optimal wellness.[5] Ally Day and I have dubbed this phenomenon "quantified healthism," pointing to the ways in which visualizing and quantifying the body become linked to moral obligations toward health:

> As our experiences of embodiment become replaced by numerical models, our alienation from our bodies grows, as does our subsequent invalidation of our self-knowledge. We no longer simply rely on professionalized clinicians and their scientific authority to explain our bodies to ourselves, but on black-boxed and proprietary software that both determines what metrics are meaningful and how to make sense of them. What cannot be quantified is dismissed. Quantified healthism is rooted in these dual forces of neoliberal self-responsibility, which confuses health with virtue, and the abdication of authority to biomedical technologies, which reduces health to the discrete and measurable.[6]

Further advancing this idea, I argue that the three technologies at the center of this analysis materialize disability through visualization and datafication, confronting (prospective) users with choices that were previously nonexistent. Embedded in a sociotechnical context rife with credibility contests, discriminatory health care practices, and ableist material and social infrastructure, disabled people and the prospective parents of disabled people are held personally accountable for managing disability through its prevention, treatment, or cure. At the same time, their experiential and embodied knowledge is questioned or dismissed outright when it comes into conflict with medical authority, a situation that essentially traps them in a double bind. Importantly, I do not believe any of the technologies or contexts I analyze here are exceptional in the pressures they apply to users; rather, they are indicative of a strengthening moral regime that demands both responsibility and compliance.

Each case presented in this book builds toward my ultimate conclusion while emphasizing a particular aspect of the tangled knowledge politics that drives medical technology design and use. Interviews with prospective parents and genetic counselors reveal the manner in which prenatal genetic testing technology reinforces the presumed relationship between knowledge acquisition and responsible parenthood—and, by extension, responsible citizenship—while simultaneously divorcing disability from the embodied experience of disabled people themselves. Interviews with recipients of deep brain stimulation and their carers, read alongside hospital guidance, highlight epistemic invalidation in pursuit of neoliberal body management. Users of do-it-yourself diabetes technologies and the community documents they create provide a counterexample that rejects the hegemonic relationship between medical professionals and submissive patients but ultimately reifies the value of self-governance and individual responsibility. Finally, drawing together insights across these cases, I argue that an increasingly technologied medical establishment reinscribes the individualization, privatization, and depoliticization of disability while at the same time casting the elimination of disability as a public good.[7] Technology users find methods of disrupting patterns of power and authority within the rigid confines of medicine. Transgressions across authoritative, knowledge, and bodily boundaries become mandatory for the survival of disabled people, as does the co-option of medical technology as a means of displacing the immense weight of ableism and personal accountability.

The contribution I make is threefold: First, by bridging the gap between rich, inductive qualitative data and disability studies, I recenter disability theory on the very real, complex, and consequential decisions made by disabled people and their prospective parents on a daily basis. Empirical work attending to embodied and experiential expertise has been sparse, despite the increasing activity of health movements devoted to challenging the assumptions of scientific and expert knowledge production.[8] This empirical qualitative study strengthens and supports the emergence of disability theory on medical technologies, confirming and nuancing tensions between embodied and clinical knowledge, the invalidation of experience, and the value of disabled knowledge practices. Second, in placing three seemingly disparate medical technologies side by side, I shift away from a perspective that views each technological innovation as exceptional and instead recognize the commonalities in their designs, practices, and discourses. Doing so is my method for giving critical analysis of technology a way to catch up to the speed of technological progress itself. By setting these medical technologies alongside one another in my analysis, I seek to demythologize them, showing that they are neither exceptional nor socially deterministic, and thus pulling these discourses and practices back into the mundane. This analysis does work to contribute to a growing set of theoretical tools that can be applied across medical technologies, allowing for ongoing consultation in the development and deployment of future technologies, rather than defaulting to reactive critique. Finally, by characterizing the tensions between personal and social responsibility, between embodied and clinical expertise, and between individual autonomy and public health models of health care, I create a scholarly foundation on which to build alternative futures.

Genes, Brains, and Pancreases

In one sense, this is a book about three technologies: prenatal genetic testing, deep brain stimulation, and artificial pancreas systems. In another sense, this is not a book about technology at all. It is instead a book about how our bodyminds shape and are shaped by the material and discursive world we inhabit, and the lived consequences of that constant remolding. It is a book about people, about power, about knowledge, with three medical technologies mediating that story, as they mediate our relationships to ourselves and each other. In this section, I provide a brief overview of each of these technologies, along with a justification for why it is an important site for thinking about disability, authority, and responsibility.

Routinizing Responsibility in Prenatal Genetic Testing

Prenatal genetic screening and testing (PGT) is a suite of technologies, strategies, and processes used to provide prospective parents with probable and diagnostic information about their own or their prospective child's genetic makeup. Clinics have used PGT since the late 1960s, with the introduction of amniocentesis.[9] Initially, PGT relied on biochemical and cytological methods for the detection of heritable metabolic and chromosomal conditions. These processes often carry with them a small risk of miscarriage, and so they were reserved only for pregnancies deemed "high risk," such as those involving a pregnant person over age thirty-five. Diagnostic tests of this nature analyze genetic material from amniotic fluid (amniocentesis), placental tissue (chorionic villus sampling), or, in the case of in vitro fertilization, the preimplantation embryo.[10] However, the development of serum testing, which requires only a blood draw, and ultrasound-dependent strategies, which pose no health risk, shifted prenatal genetic technologies into routine obstetric care. Thus emerged prenatal genetic "screening," which provides information about probable risk rather than definitive diagnosis.[11] Common screening procedures include carrier screening, which makes predictions based on the prospective parents' genetic information; nuchal translucency screening, which interprets measurements of the fetus via ultrasound; and quad screening, which measures the pregnant person's blood for substances linked to conditions including Down syndrome, Edwards syndrome, and neural tube defects.[12] Findings from screenings are typically confirmed through more invasive diagnostic procedures.

If the debut of amniocentesis in the 1960s marks one transformation in prenatal care, the deployment of cell-free DNA (cfDNA) screening in the early 2010s marks another. Alternatively called noninvasive prenatal screening (NIPS), this technique tests fetal DNA circulating in the blood of the expectant parent. With very little health risk to parent or fetus and the ability to screen for a wide array of chromosomal conditions, NIPS has flourished in clinical practice. As Gareth Thomas and colleagues note, this new, ostensibly less risky, modality has intensified concerns around informed consent, conceptions of disability, commercialization, and routinization.[13] At the time of this writing, no known studies have been conducted to determine what proportion of pregnant people receive some kind of genetic screening or testing, though the American College of Obstetricians and Gynecologists recommends that screening and diagnostic testing be offered to all pregnant people. It is reasonable to assume that the majority of prospective parents in the United States are at least presented with the option to pursue some form of prenatal genetic screening or testing as part of standard obstetric care.[14] We do not yet know how *Dobbs v. Jackson Women's Health Organization,* the 2022 U.S. Supreme Court case that overturned the constitutional right to abortion, will transform the delivery of prenatal screening and testing in the future. As of 2022, fourteen U.S. states had restrictions that, if they allowed termination at all, allowed it only very early in a pregnancy, before diagnostic tests like amniocentesis are possible, and seven had restrictions on pregnancy termination on the basis of fetal genetic conditions.[15] How these policies may evolve, and what that could mean for clinical experiences of prenatal screening and testing, remains to be seen.

As genetic information proliferated through modern obstetrics, a need arose for professionals to interpret and mediate the delivery of that information. Enter genetic counselors.[16] Sitting at the nexus of medical genetics and psychology, genetic counselors occupy a role distinct from obstetricians in both training and practice, "mobiliz[ing] observations of genetic anomalies as the basis of new medical conditions, organizations, and personal identities."[17] They are specialists who work in a wide variety of settings, including hospitals, private clinics, academic institutions, and commercial genetic testing labs. Established as a field of practice as early as 1947, genetic counseling was at first conducted primarily by medical geneticists—doctors by training—and was explicitly directive and eugenic. Soon, however, genetic counselors formed a professional class distinct from geneticists, and with that differentiation came an approach that privileged individual choice over public health policy.[18] With this pivot, genetic counseling adopted a rhetoric of "nondirective" care, demanding that "professionals should not present any reproductive decision as 'correct' or advantageous for a person or society."[19] However, some observers—such as Gareth Thomas, who examined Down syndrome screening in the United Kingdom—have argued that the integration of genetic screening into routine care is itself directive.[20] Further, others have called for an explicit interrogation of how disability is discussed in the context of genetic counseling, in part to refute accusations that the presence of screening fosters the belief that congenital disability is something that should be avoided.[21] While genetic counselors are cast as experts of genetic information in the clinic, most pregnant people currently receive prenatal genetic screening and testing without encountering a genetic counselor at all. Genetic counseling is typically recommended for pregnant people who receive atypical screening or test results, have a familial history of genetic differences, or have a pregnancy otherwise categorized as risky. Most others receive screening and test results directly through their clinicians or through an online portal linked to a commercial genetic testing lab.

Of the three cases I examine in this book, prenatal screening and diagnosis has most thoroughly penetrated traditional medical care. The technologies of PGT represent an institutionalized form of medical surveillance that interacts with issues of gendered labor and the geneticization of disability.[22] Disability studies scholars have written at length about the connections between prenatal genetic testing and the elimination of disability, with Rosemarie Garland-Thomson calling PGT a form of "velvet eugenics," which "seems like common sense, yet . . . hides its violence and inequality behind claims of patient autonomy and under a veil of voluntary consent."[23] PGT exemplifies perceived tensions between disability and reproductive rights, as well as individual choice models of health care, which assume a prospective parent has autonomy over reproductive choices, and public health models, which implement screening technologies in order to forestall costly public health expenditures on the care of nonnormative bodyminds.[24] Further, this case study explores the social, political, and ethical complexities of pregnancy management, in which the nonnormative bodymind in question is both within and distinct from the pregnant person, and simultaneously real as a fetus and imagined as a future child. Disability is both materialized through the visualization techniques of PGT and dematerialized by the way the disability diagnosis is divorced from the embodied experience of currently living disabled people. While I have gestured to a rich history of critical scholarship analyzing prenatal genetic testing, PGT has rarely been considered in conversation with other medical technologies; instead, it has been treated as exceptional and anomalous in its ethical and cultural implications. By placing PGT alongside other medical devices and processes, I show that its implications are not exceptional, but merely one manifestation of the neoliberal pressures bearing down on disabled bodyminds.

The Limits of Agency in Deep Brain Stimulation

Humans have been conducting brain surgery for all of recorded history. Up to a tenth of all analyzed skulls from the Neolithic period show signs of trepanation, an early surgical procedure involving drilling a hole in the skull.[25] Ancient and premodern physicians, including Hippocrates (fifth century BCE) and Abu Al Qasim Al Zahrawi (tenth century AD), documented interventions for traumatic brain injuries and neurological conditions, many of which serve as the basis for modern techniques.[26] Beginning in the sixteenth century, advancements in anatomical scholarship and surgical methods paved the way for modern neurosurgery.[27]

While informed by these histories, the practice of deep brain stimulation can be traced to a single development in the early twentieth century: stereotactic surgery. Using a three-dimensional coordinate system to target key areas of the brain, and enabled by the use of a metal cage attached to the skull of the person undergoing surgery, stereotaxy both extended the possibilities of neurosurgery and greatly reduced mortality rates.[28] In the 1930s, Canadian surgeon Wilder Graves Penfield piloted the "Montreal procedure," a technique that used direct cortical stimulation to map the brain. Initially used for ablation as an intervention for epilepsy, this method of mapping and detection was soon applied to acute and long-term stimulation procedures for psychiatric and motor conditions.[29] One such use was for Parkinson's disease, a progressive condition that affects the nervous system, resulting in issues with movement, including tremor, stiffness, and balance problems.[30] In 1968, the introduction of levodopa, a precursor to dopamine now commonly used as a medication to manage the motor symptoms of Parkinson's, led to a decline in stereotactic surgeries.[31] That same year, however, the first implantable neurostimulator came to market. Initially developed by Minneapolis-based medical technology company Medtronic in the 1960s for heart conditions, by the 1970s, stimulators were being used for a wide range of neurological and psychiatric conditions, from epilepsy to schizophrenia to movement disorders.[32] It was not until the late 1990s and early 2000s, however, that the U.S. Food and Drug Administration (FDA) approved any neurostimulation technique as standard treatment, and even then, these approvals extended only to Parkinson's tremor, advanced Parkinson's, dystonia, and essential tremor.[33] The FDA approved DBS for epilepsy in 2018 and has approved a Humanitarian Device Exemption (HDE) for the use of DBS for obsessive-compulsive disorder.[34] DBS continues to be trialed for a wide range of uses, including as an intervention for major depressive disorder, chronic pain, Tourette's syndrome, autism spectrum conditions, and self-injurious behavior.[35]

The modern deep brain stimulator is a surgical implant delivering electrical impulses to targeted areas of the brain. The clinician first develops a three-dimensional image, CT scan, or MRI of the recipient's brain to determine the electrode placement. Next, in a surgery during which the recipient is typically awake, the clinician inserts electrodes, also known as leads, through a small hole drilled in the skull. The clinician tests the electrode placement by posing questions to the recipient or walking the person through a series of exercises.[36] The leads are then connected to wires that run to an internal pulse generator (IPG) implanted in the chest, which powers the electrodes.[37] Depending on the intended use and the recipient, electrodes may be implanted on one side of the brain or both sides, powered by one or two IPGs.

We do not know the precise mechanism by which DBS works. The American Association of Neurological Surgeons posits: "DBS is presumed to help modulate dysfunctional circuits in the brain so that the brain can function more effectively. This is accomplished by sending continuous electrical signals to specific target areas of the brain, which block impulses that cause neurological dysfunctions."[38] The rather unclear mechanism by which DBS works contributes to some uncertainty about whether it will improve target symptoms in any given person. Following implantation, the recipient works with a care team to program the device, a process of adjusting levels of stimulation that can take anywhere from several months to years. Deep brain stimulation does not cure any condition; rather, it is intended to mitigate and manage symptoms. If the system is turned off, dies, or otherwise does not operate, symptoms will reemerge.

Interrogating invasive and complex biotechnological interventions like DBS leads to new insights about agency, responsibility, and disability. First, previous research suggests that user education and participation in decision-making are not prioritized in the context of medical implants.[39] Further, interventions that address neurological and psychiatric conditions can result in side effects that have impacts on thinking and feeling, such as personality changes, emergent mental health issues, and self-estrangement, necessitating attention to the balance between clinical outcomes and potential harms.[40] Additionally, rhetorics of restoration, control, and autonomy characterize the contexts in which DBS is adopted, yet in reality, continued medical surveillance, technological dependence, and unmet expectations temper these promises.[41] This case study offers an opportunity to explore what John Gardner describes as "a conviction in technology-oriented solutions, a drive to alleviate suffering, a suspicion of commercial interests, doubts over the ability of regulatory initiatives, and anxiety over a precarious future."[42] Finally, the manner in which nonnormative bodyminds and disabling symptoms are identified, standardized, and made legible in order for individuals to become eligible for DBS—and the symptoms deemed important to mitigate through DBS—offer a site to interrogate how disability becomes operationalized in medical technology, and what elements of embodiment are delegitimated in that process.

Taking Control with DIY Artificial Pancreas Systems

Identified as early as 1500 BCE, diabetes mellitus is a condition in which cells cannot use glucose properly to produce energy because of issues with the body's production or use of the pancreatic hormone insulin.[43] This results in high levels of blood glucose, which can damage blood vessels and organs and cause the buildup of blood acids called ketones. Without intervention, this buildup can lead to death.

Prior to the 1921 discovery of insulin by Frederick Banting, Charles Best, James Bertram Collip, and John MacLeod, a diabetes mellitus diagnosis often came with a very short life expectancy.[44] Their discovery, and the successful injection of beef pancreatic extract into fourteen-year-old Leonard Thompson the following year, marks a shift from diabetes as death sentence to diabetes as chronic illness. While physicians as early as the fifth century noted at least two variants of diabetes, it was not until 1936 that British scientist Harold Himsworth differentiated between diabetes that responded to insulin treatment and typically appeared in childhood (subsequently dubbed "type 1") and diabetes that was resistant to insulin treatment, typically appearing in adulthood (type 2).[45] While these categories are not without contention, this naming convention, along with type 1.5, which bears a resemblance to type 1 but is usually undetected until adulthood, dominates modern diabetes discourse. In this book, I examine technologies developed for insulin-sensitive (type 1/type 1.5) diabetes.

In the century following insulin's isolation, technological innovations have targeted two key processes: monitoring blood glucose and administering insulin. Early monitoring techniques, involving urine test strips, tablets, and dipsticks, focused on measuring ketone levels in urine as a proxy for blood glucose. These tools gave way to blood glucose test strips, initially developed in 1965 for clinical use only.[46] By the early 1980s, portable glucose monitors entered the market, meaning people with T1D could test their blood glucose at home.[47] In 1999, the Food and Drug Administration approved the first continuous glucose monitor (CGM), a device that uses a disposable sensor to detect glucose levels in the interstitial fluid at regular intervals. By 2019, approximately 30 percent of the more than 22,000 people in the T1D Exchange registry reported using CGMs, although there are significant disparities in access to and use of CGMs by race.[48] Modern monitoring tools offer on-demand access to blood glucose levels by interfacing with devices such as mobile phones and smart watches, enabling a level of precision management that was previously unimaginable.

The other key process, insulin delivery, can be accomplished through several means. Long- and rapid-acting insulin can be injected manually several times throughout the day, a regimen called multiple daily injections (MDI). While subcutaneous syringes are commonly used, since the early 1980s, MDI users have also been able to opt for preloaded insulin pens. Alternatively, beginning in the 1990s, subcutaneous insulin infusion through insulin pumps became widely available. Typically injecting insulin via a cannula that the user replaces every few days, these programmable devices can deliver insulin continuously.[49] While MDI remains the most common approach to insulin delivery for people with T1D, there were approximately 400,000 pump users in the United States as of 2018.[50] Notably, until very recently, blood glucose monitoring and insulin delivery were always independent processes, with the user interpreting blood glucose results and manually determining insulin dosages. The increasing portability and usability of diabetes technologies means that the majority of management has moved outside the clinic. As self-management became possible through technologies for glucose monitoring and insulin delivery, users became increasingly responsible for outcomes. Consequently, discourses of blame, noncompliance, and personal responsibility proliferate in modern diabetes care.

Do-it-yourself artificial pancreas systems (DIYAPS) can be characterized as both a set of techniques and a social movement. Sometimes called hybrid closed-loop or automated delivery systems, DIYAPS controls insulin delivery with limited user input by linking a CGM, an insulin pump, a smartphone or smart watch, and open-source algorithms.[51] Using current and historical CGM data and user input to administer insulin automatically, DIYAPS effectively "closes the loop" between glucose monitoring and insulin delivery. Some variants include additional hardware components, such as a microcomputer or a device used to bridge Bluetooth-enabled devices to other components. Currently, three DIYAPS variants are in regular use: OpenAPS, AndroidAPS, and Loop.[52] OpenAPS was the first widely reproducible DIY hybrid closed loop, initially developed by Dana Lewis, Ben West, and Scott Leibrand in the United States in 2015.[53] It was based in part on a design that Lewis and Leibrand began working on in 2013. It is compatible with some Medtronic pumps (older pumps with a security feature that allows communication with other devices) and uses a microcomputer and an optional smart watch. OpenAPS enacts changes in insulin delivery by referring to trends in data such as insulin sensitivity factor (ISF), basal rates, and carbohydrate ratios.[54] Nate Racklyeft and Pete Schwamb, also in the United States, developed Loop in 2015 using a different algorithm and set of hardware requirements. It is compatible with additional insulin pumps, such as the tubeless Omnipod, and uses an iPhone, Apple Watch, and RileyLink, a specially designed communication component named after Schwamb's daughter with T1D.[55] Milos Kozak and Adrian Tappe, of the Czech Republic and Austria, respectively, followed with AndroidAPS. Modeled after and using the same algorithm as OpenAPS, AndroidAPS utilizes Android technology and is compatible with a large selection of pumps (including Dana R, Dana RS, Roche Combo, Roche Insight, and Virtual Pump), making it more accessible to European users. While DIYAPS automates some management, Lewis notes that the DIY community works actively to address misconceptions that artificial pancreas systems are technological cures rather than tools requiring active attention and engagement.[56] Both clinicians and members of the DIY community have expressed concerns that DIYAPS will result in the deskilling of people newly diagnosed with T1D, making it more difficult for them to use more traditional insulin pump systems or MDI if needed.[57] To counteract the myth of full automation, the term "hybrid closed loop" is often used to clarify user engagement. With "closed loop" modified by "hybrid," this term suggests a less autonomous technology. For example, a DIYAPS user will continue to do a bolus (a dose of insulin) manually to account for eating.

DIYAPS is a bridge between the DIY bio and health social movements. "DIY bio" refers to an undefined field of practice with its roots in citizen science, hacking, and the maker movement. Broadly adhering to a "hacker ethic," it is characterized by decentralization, collaboration, and access, with an aim toward social betterment.[58] Health social movements, particularly embodied health movements, challenge hegemonic science and medicine through experience of illness or disability.[59] Christopher Kelty notes that members of the DIY bio movement are largely concerned with issues of legitimacy and credibility as they challenge the hegemony of elite scientific authority, resisting the preoccupation with economic productivity that characterizes "Big Bio" (biology as practiced in universities, corporations, and governmental projects) in favor of an approach that embraces the "demystification and democratization of science."[60] This is an ethos shared by the DIYAPS community. The DIY community also marks a departure from traditional knowledge-building and knowledge-sharing activities in research communities. As DIYAPS contributors Dana Lewis and Scott Leibrand write: "The user community has valuable insight, data, and experiences that can help everyone (device manufacturers, health care providers, and users) to build better tools to better manage life with diabetes."[61] Self-determination and individual responsibility are central to DIYAPS. Therefore, the DIYAPS movement (which often appears online using the hashtag #WeAreNotWaiting) also provides a powerful site to think through knowledge production and experiential expertise. When considering a topic area in which scientific expertise has historically trumped embodied knowledge—and credibility to speak about disability has been predicated on membership within a medical elite—it is necessary to deconstruct ideas around knowledge and truth to understand how systemic power imbalances and epistemic injustice have marginalized disabled people in their own lives, and how resistance movements such as DIYAPS transform those knowledge practices.[62]

Methodological Notes

At the center of this work are three sets of interviews. I conducted semistructured and unstructured interviews with forty-one informants over the course of two and a half years.[63] Informants included medical technology users and secondary informants; the composition of the latter groups varied by case.[64] Notably, the methodology used in the case discussing PGT strategically puts the perspectives of users and clinicians in conversation, as it focuses narrowly on the clinical interaction of engaging with PGT, while the other two cases are concerned exclusively with users and their communities. The scope of this research is primarily the U.S. health care system, although the globalization of health care and the democratization of the Internet trouble these boundaries. Informants often engaged in cross-national dialogues, gathering information online from around the world. All informants in both the PGT and DBS cases lived in the United States. Several DIYAPS informants resided in Europe. The DIY community is dispersed, existing mostly in online spaces that cross borders and oceans. While there are some distinctions in the health care systems in which users operate, the shift to agential actor outside the compliant patient role and the construction of personal and collective responsibility in DIY spaces carried across geographic boundaries.

During the same period when I was conducting interviews, I collected and analyzed user-directed documents such as fact sheets, promotional materials, and user-created guidance.[65] I obtained documents from an eclectic array of sources, including hospital and health care systems, commercial medical technology manufacturers, online blogs and community forums, and regulatory agencies. I understand these documents not as communicating facts, but as artifacts as value laden and enmeshed in credibility contests as the technologies they describe. As such, I analyzed them similarly to and in conversation with informant interviews.

My analytical framework, along with my epistemological position as described in chapter 1, is scavenged from across disciplines and practices.[66] My analysis is inductive, always hewing closely to the words and lives of my informants. I appreciate the space to explore context, ambiguity, and pluralism offered by inductive frameworks broadly. I seek in my analysis an epistemological openness and humility, deriving themes from informants' experiences in an iterative manner. I draw broadly from the processes of grounded theory but establish no universalizing theory, instead leaning into contextual understandings.[67] I draw also from hermeneutical phenomenology, which allows me to both value my informants' experiential knowledge and contextualize it alongside the factors that mediate their interpretations.[68] In this way, I can uphold personal insights as legitimate sources of knowledge while equally recognizing that those insights are filtered through historical contexts and hegemonic discourses. Such a patchwork approach, sometimes dubbed "generic qualitative analysis," has been identified as particularly useful when applied to new fields, which aligns with my goal of blending several fields of theory and practice in order to gain new insights and generate alternatives to the epistemologies, processes, and practices that currently drive the development and deployment of medical technologies.[69] Generic qualitative approaches allow for a methodological playfulness that "support[s] new fields of research, theoretical perspectives, new questions, or new approaches to old research problems."[70]

Writing about and interpreting the emotional and experiential realities of the informants who contribute to this book—many of whom are disabled or chronically ill—comes with its own ethical demands. As a feminist researcher, I grapple with issues of representation and interpretation. Knowledge production is, by its nature, a communal event; in the context of research, Caroline Ramazanoglu and Janet Holland describe it as a negotiation among researcher, subject, and epistemic communities.[71] I am accountable to all of the communities with which I engage throughout this work. As such, I am particularly attentive to the historical and contemporary subjugation of marginalized people in the pursuit of Western scientific inquiry.[72] Therefore, I strive to produce work that is neither extractive nor oppressive and creates space for people to be active producers of their own interpretations. Informants had opportunities to review and revise their initial transcripts, request follow-up interviews, and comment on an early draft of this monograph.[73] These transcript and draft reviews were precipitated less by my desire to ensure the accuracy of the interviews, as might be the case in a study using an objectivist epistemology, than by my resolve to ensure that informants felt the transcripts and findings resonated with their experiences. In this way, the informants were active participants in constructing and reconstructing the narratives that underpin this work.[74]

Chapter Overview

In chapter 1, "The Acceptable Bodymind in a Technologied World," I put critical disability studies, feminist science and technology studies, and medical sociology in conversation to understand how Western biomedicine became a field animated by a moral imperative to intervene on bodily difference through technological means. I argue that five critical insights are necessary for understanding the new epistemic, ontological, and moral regimes enabled by an increasing reliance on technoscience in medicine:

1. Disability is a permeable category.
2. Ableism and neoliberalism are mutually implicated.
3. Medicalization matters.
4. Technology is not neutral.
5. Embodiment and experience are legitimate sources of knowledge.

In chapter 2, "Becoming Responsible with Prenatal Genetic Testing," I explore the seamless integration of prenatal genetic screening and testing into routine medical care, the production of medical knowledge, and the relationship between knowledge accumulation and an assumption of responsible parenting. An analysis of interviews with prospective parents and genetic counselors and user-directed guidance documents illustrates a clear relationship between social perceptions of responsible parenthood and an obligation to pursue testing. Deference to medical authority, however, creates a context in which acquiring "too much" knowledge represents a transgression that jeopardizes the peace of mind ostensibly acquired through screening. I also consider the rigid binaries on which disability is constructed in the clinic—physiological/social, inspiration/tragedy—and their impacts on clinical trust and the meaning of informed consent. Paired with an illusion of scientific certainty enabled through the visualization and materialization of disability as solely and discretely located in extra chromosomes or translocated segments, PGT disallows embodied experiences of disability as knowledge contributions. Ultimately, this chapter exposes perceptions of the obligatory nature of screening and testing in pursuit of responsible parenthood and tensions between the knowledge sought by prospective parents and the information proffered by professionals.

Chapter 3, "Losing and Taking Control with Deep Brain Stimulation," examines the use of DBS techniques for neurological and movement conditions such as Parkinson's disease and essential tremor. This analysis links the design, use, and discourse around deep brain stimulation to the understanding of disability as a purely physiological phenomenon in need of medical intervention, albeit one resulting in social stigma. Once disability is firmly located within the individual, perceptions of personal responsibility to manage it emerge as central to decision-making, especially when elements of disability are observable, such as tremor, or impede economic or social productivity. Additionally, DBS users experience epistemic invalidation or dismissal when their embodiment challenges clinical authority in some way, often through the experience of physical, neurological, or psychiatric symptoms related to either the precipitating condition or their implants. Beyond these individual instances of invalidation, this case also makes clear a discrepancy in how disability and invasiveness are understood by users, clinicians, and device manufacturers. Some users understand DBS as less invasive than the surveillance and side effects of medication or the stigma of observable disability, contradicting clinical guidelines. Drawing on personal accounts of deep brain stimulation and on the narratives produced in user-directed guidance documents, this case emphasizes the relationship between medical intervention and neoliberal body management, as well as the consequences of embodied knowledge that challenges or resists medical authority. I argue that while deep brain stimulation operates under a rhetoric of empowerment and control, that control is ultimately restricted both by epistemic invalidation of embodied experience in the clinic and by systemic pressures of neoliberal ableism and compulsory able-bodiedness.

The third case study, chapter 4, "Reimagining Agency with Do-It-Yourself Artificial Pancreas Systems," examines DIY diabetes technology as a site of opportunity to reframe expertise and authority in medicine. The DIY community represents both an active challenge to the submissive patient role expected under medical authority and a reification of self-responsibility. Drawing from interviews with users—both those who developed DIY systems for themselves and parents or guardians who developed them for their young children—as well as guidance documents produced by and for DIYers, this analysis highlights a particular manifestation of personal and collective responsibility that arises from invalidation by the medical establishment and the failure of regulated management options to attend to the lived realities of diabetes. Further, the DIY community directly resists and challenges medical authority through the explicit endorsement of experiential community-based knowledge. While ostensibly animated by a community ethos that endorses transparency, collaboration, and access, this message is in tension with the profiles of successful DIYers—educated, self-motivated, knowledgeable—revealing an internalization of the principles of neoliberal body management that reinscribe self-governance and individual responsibility. Ultimately, this case exemplifies a resistance to the passive patient role that characterizes medical authority, asserting disabled knowledge as a force to destabilize hegemonic power relations.

In the book's Conclusion, I draw together these three case studies to demonstrate that there is no way to exist in a nonnormative body without transgressing the boundaries of medical authority or the boundaries of what constitutes an acceptable bodymind. Attempts to politicize disabled embodiment are met with pressures to further individualize and privatize interventions, retrenching the authority of the medical establishment. Disabled people and their prospective parents are often confronted with a double bind: being held personally accountable for disability while simultaneously having their embodied, experiential, or practical expertise invalidated in favor of medical authority. This context is further complicated by medical understandings of and expectations for disability that are directly in tension with the embodied understandings of users. Clinicians perceive disabled people's assertions of embodied knowledge as transgression. Strained communication, dissatisfaction, and trauma become common in medical settings, often resulting in the development of support communities, where informal knowledge exchanges occur outside medical jurisdiction. I argue that medical technology users imagine a new, more liberatory knowledge politic within this constraining sociotechnical system, one in which individual autonomy is traded for collective experience, embodied knowledge is embraced, and the boundaries of bodily integrity and knowledge authority are challenged. Finally, I resist a techno-deterministic narrative, arguing that medical technologies take on an ambivalent role in these situations, representing both hegemonic authority demanding closer approximation to the ideal bodymind and an opportunity to displace the burden of neoliberal ableism. I end by calling for more explicit recognition of the social and political complexities mediated through medical technologies and by imagining a future where such technologies intervene not on nonnormative bodyminds but on the ableist infrastructures that disenfranchise them.

« 1 »

The Acceptable Bodymind in a Technologied World

Since the mid-twentieth century, American medicine has increasingly relied on technoscience for the identification, prevention, and elimination of disability. With this new mode of care came new epistemic, ontological, and moral regimes. The construction of disability as a biological phenomenon inside an increasingly technologied health care system produces social, political, and physical pressures that cede authority to medical professionals and processes, marginalizing and invalidating knowledge systems that imagine disability otherwise.

From the half century of empirical and theoretical work that has characterized this evolution, I tease out five key insights foundational to my understanding and interpretation of the cases I analyze in this book. I take time to lay out these insights and trace their intellectual origins for two reasons. First, the inductive approach I adopt for the next several chapters is one that intentionally hews closely to the interviews and documents I analyze. While I reject the notion that inductive findings emerge from data in the absence of interpretation, I also resist overabstracting or overdetermining lived experience. I wish instead to engage closely with the complexities and ambiguities of embodiment and experience in the following chapters. This necessitates explicitly laying out my epistemological position here. Second, my academic practice is rooted in inter-, cross-, and antidisciplinary approaches. I build my work on an eclectic foundation that I hope to make legible to readers through these insights. I am deeply concerned with who is considered expert and under what conditions, and as such, I strive to make apparent the diverse sets of knowledge and experience that inform my analytical perspective. The five insights explored in turn below are drawn primarily from disability studies, feminist science and technology studies, and sociology. Importantly, I aim to draw out the resonances across these fields, which are not often put into conversation with one another. In doing so, I contribute to building generative cross-disciplinary practices.

Disability Is a Permeable Category

The first insight I carry into this study holds that the meanings and ontologies of disability are situated, fluid, and multiple. As Simi Linton writes, disability is "not simply the variations that exist in human behavior, appearance, functioning, sensory acuity, and cognitive processing but, more crucially, the meaning we make of those variations."[1] Cultural, social, and political frameworks influence how and when human difference consolidates into disability. Disability is neither just a physiological fact nor a cultural artifact; it is both simultaneously, coproduced and coproducing. The "line that we draw between the biological and the social . . . is artificial," Susan Wendell states, arguing that nonnormative bodyminds can be understood only as resulting from the complex interaction between the two.[2] Therefore, how disabled and nonnormative bodyminds become legible in health care systems is a social and political question as much as a scientific one.

Thus, there is no one universal experience of disability, nor are there definitive bodily characteristics that innately cohere to produce disability. Further, disability can be understood as many different things in a single historical and geographic moment; emergent understandings do not necessarily obscure or eliminate older knowledge systems or framing conventions. Disability studies scholars refer to these framing conventions as "models." Schemas for understanding disability, models expose and shape social values and pathways to epistemic authority, determining what disability means in part through who has the authority to define it. Erving Goffman's work on the framing of social categories and phenomena suggests that the organizing of experiences is not innate but informed by complex social and political processes.[3] The frame through which disability is understood—produced and producing certain social, political, and material realities—creates conditions under which certain people and groups have categorical authority to produce knowledge about disability. Explicating frames is a valuable practice, in that it "allows us to see that events do not in and of themselves dictate the pathways along which public responses will move."[4] In the context of medicine, we can then push back against the taken-for-grantedness of detection and cure as natural responses to bodily and cognitive difference. Making explicit the competing knowledge systems that construct disability allows me to examine how and where invalidated or illegitimate embodied knowledge might inform medical technology and practice.

One of the oldest recognized models of disability is one that frames it as a moral failure or spiritual challenge. Under this model, moral authorities such as clergy define when nonnormativity becomes disability, determine its causes (such as parental failure to abide by social mores), and prescribe the appropriate intervention (such as exorcism or abandonment). In Western societies, religious and moral models, particularly those emerging from Christian traditions, have long determined authority over disability.[5] However, the twentieth century and the dawn of modernity marked a decline in the influence of religion in everyday life. While disability is now less often understood through religious frameworks, the links between morality and normativity remain tightly entwined. Health is conflated with righteousness; its absence is viewed as a moral failing.[6]

The gap in authority over disability that was produced by religion's declining influence was rapidly filled by the professionalization of medicine and the emergence of a class of medical experts.[7] Social progress and the common good became explicitly linked to rationality and scientific progress.[8] With the rise of professional clinicians, intricate gatekeeping processes and systems of epistemic privilege emerged in which disabled bodyminds became not just objects of personal responsibility, as in the moralization of disability under a moral model, but objects of social control. In part, this control came from the power to categorize, name, and intervene on nonnormativity-cum-pathology. Thus, as secularization and modernization reduced the influence of religion as a governing force, the individual (or medical) model became the dominant interpretation of disability. This model privileges individualistic, biomedical explanations for disability, asserting that disability has biological origins and is located solely in the body. Disability is discrete, identifiable, and treatable through scientific and medical regimens. Salient to this model is the construction of a normal/abnormal binary, in which able-bodiedness and able-mindedness are fetishized.[9] The model intrinsically encompasses the social idealization of bodyminds as "young, strong, healthy," pathologizing any embodiment falling outside those fictive norms.[10]

Accompanying these ideals is what Alison Kafer calls the "curative imaginary," which "not only *expects* and *assumes* intervention, but also cannot imagine or comprehend anything other than intervention."[11] Medicine as a practice has enabled many disabled people to live or to live with greater quality of life, but it has also forced an understanding of disability as solely biological or physiological—and therefore deeply individualized. Further, with the development of medical technologies that can treat, manage, or identify disability, a transfiguration of moral responsibility as taken place. For example, in most contemporary societies, congenital disability may no longer be read as a result of the lax moral standards of the parents, but not identifying or managing pregnancy through prenatal genetic screening is often understood as irresponsible or immoral parenting.[12] As discussed below, this understanding of disability both informs and is informed by the social demand for neoliberal personal responsibility.

In direct response to the oppressive nature of the medical model, disabled activists in the mid-twentieth century began advocating for a model rooted in social construction. By some accounts originating with the UK-based Union of the Physically Impaired Against Segregation (UPIAS) in the 1970s, the social model argues that physical or biological differences—referred to as impairments—are not disabling in and of themselves. Rather, disability emerges through social exclusion, physical inaccessibility, and attitudinal barriers. Disability, thus, is "something imposed on top of our impairments, by the way we are unnecessarily isolated and excluded from full participation in society."[13] The social model is concerned with "barrier removal, anti-discrimination legislation, independent living, and other responses to social oppression."[14] This model has since come to signal alignment with disability rights. It has been an extremely effective political orientation that has enabled significant policy and infrastructural changes across the world.

However, recent scholarship poses a challenge to the social model. First, as Tom Shakespeare writes, the model "so strongly disowns individual and medical approaches that it risks implying that impairment is not a problem," thus invalidating the experiences of people who live with pain or other disabling phenomena that cannot be directly linked to social oppression.[15] Further, the social model of disability does not attend to what Moya Bailey and Izetta Mobley refer to as the "particular vulnerability of Black, women, and gender-nonconforming bodies," refusing to authorize individual desire for treatment that for many has been consistently denied. "As uncomfortable as it may make those of us engaged in the Disability Studies field," they write, "some communities are actually yearning for not only care but treatment and cure. Part of corporeal autonomy as a theoretical stance—one that links both Blackness and disability—is that it allows for people to choose what is best for their bodies: treatment, cure, or a resistance to medical intervention altogether."[16] Finally, the social model assumes that a universally designed environment could eliminate disability as a social category—a claim that is both curiously curative and erroneous, as it does not take into account the heterogeneity of disability.

As disability studies cohered as a field in the late twentieth and early twenty-first century, additional models for understanding disability emerged. Tobin Siebers's conception of complex embodiment ameliorates the tensions between the social and medical models by recognizing the social and political dimensions of disability as real and significant, while also not dismissing the biological, physiological, and material impacts of disability. Siebers writes that particular embodied experiences of chronic pain, aging, and other health effects

> are neither less significant than disability caused by the environment nor to be considered defects or deviations merely because they are resistant to change. Rather, they belong to the spectrum of human variation, conceived both as variability between individuals and as variability within an individual's lifecycle, and they need to be considered in tandem with social forces affecting disability.[17]

Kafer reconceptualizes disability as a political/relational object, which serves to denaturalize and repoliticize it as a "potential site of cultural imaginings."[18] Under this paradigm, disability is not constrained by the material or discursive models that preceded it, but is a political object with enough interpretive flexibility to encourage coalition building. The "relational" aspect of this frame also allows for individual lived experiences to shape interpretations of disability; such an approach counters the social model's perceived condemnation of individual desire for medical intervention.

In this work, I strive to make explicit the many competing, resonating, and conflicting framings of disability that are constantly interacting in the clinical space. Epistemologically, however, I pay particular attention to the imbrication of the material and the discursive, as exemplified by Kafer and Siebers. As explained below, this attention is imperative, given my assumptions about the agency and influence of materiality on epistemological realities. We are shaped by our material world even as we are shaping it. The availability of medical technologies and their material consequences fundamentally affects the decisions that can be made and the moral weight of each option.

Ableism and Neoliberalism Are Mutually Implicated

Key to understanding the double bind of responsibility and epistemic invalidation facing disabled people in the clinic is reckoning with who holds authority and responsibility to name and manage disability. To do so, I must first acknowledge the social conditions that determine disability as a phenomenon in need of management. Ableism is a consequence of classifying disability as an individualized, medical, and curable phenomenon. Further, as I argue, ableism is an integral part of the complex context in which people choose to pursue medical intervention. It is impossible to consider medical devices and the pressure to adopt them without first considering how and when the bodymind is considered deviant and in need of intervention.

Taking for granted that disability is not a stable material condition of the body, it becomes clear that disability as a category can exist only in relation to its counterpart, ability. The manifestation of these poles necessarily produces a preference for one of them—in this case, ability. Siebers dubs this preference the "ideology of ability," which is "at its simplest, the preference for able-bodiedness. At its most radical, it defines the baseline by which humanness is determined, setting the measure of body and mind that gives or denies human status to individual persons."[19] Other scholars refer to this preference as "ableism." According to disabled bioethicist Gregor Wolbring, ableism is characterized by

> a favoritism for certain abilities that are projected as essential by individuals, households, communities, groups, sectors, regions, countries, and cultures, while labeling real or perceived deviation from or lack of these essential abilities as a diminished state of being often leading to the accompanying disablism, the discriminatory, oppressive, or abusive behavior of oneself by others arising from the belief that people without these "essential" abilities are inferior.[20]

While ableism in some form has existed across time, today's particular type of ableism is deeply intertwined with neoliberalism. In strictly economic terms, the philosophy of neoliberalism is concerned with the deregulation and privatization of markets, the reduction of government oversight, and the expansion of the private sector into social, economic, and political life. In practice, neoliberalism is characterized by a preoccupation with individual autonomy, "global inequality, economic disparity, growth of unemployment, social exclusion, environmental destruction, and cultural homogeneity."[21] In Dan Goodley's words, it is "capitalism's global hegemonic domination."[22] The functioning of the neoliberal market hinges on the availability of economically productive and self-governing citizens. Thus, disabled people are subject to scrutiny and moral judgment. As such, in contemporary Western societies, Goodley argues, disability is produced in a context of "neoliberal ableism," which is characterized in part by "increased expectations placed on the autonomy of self-responsible individual citizens to care, educate and govern themselves."[23] The "able" bodymind is defined by its productivity, and responsible citizenship demands self-regulation and intervention when the body mind falls short. Goodley suggests that under a neoliberal ableist paradigm, a "valued citizen" is one who is

> cognitively, socially and emotionally able and competent. Biologically and psychologically stable, genetically and hormonally sound and ontologically responsible. Hearing, mobile, seeing, walking. Normal: sane, autonomous, self-sufficient, self-governing, reasonable, law-abiding and economically viable.

> White, heterosexual, male, adult, breeder, living in towns, global citizen of WENA [Western Europe, North America].[24]

As Merri Lisa Johnson and Robert McRuer observe about both social and political pressures and consequences of bodily accountability, "The decision to be capable . . . is a winding road of self-deprivation presented as a cultural good."[25] Richard Devlin and Dianne Pothier engage more substantially with a disability politics that addresses the power imbalances to which nonnormative bodyminds are subject in public life. They coin the term "dis-citizen" to signify the "system of deep, structural economic, social, political, and cultural inequality in which persons with disabilities experience unequal citizenship."[26] This regime assumes that a full citizen must be fully *productive,* where productivity is both legible to and in service of the state. They argue that dis-citizenship can never be compatible with inclusion, as "efficiency and productivity are irretrievably ableist discourses that can only condemn (some) people with disabilities to a presumptive inferior status."[27] Bailey and Mobley further nuance the differential application of citizenship across intersections of race, class, gender, and ability: "Much of the Black experience is shaped by an understanding of Black bodies as a productive labor force, leaving little room for an identity-based approach to disability. Figurations of Blackness as hyper able and yet fundamentally 'crippled' by race have been used to produce Black people as ineligible or unsound for citizenship."[28]

Under neoliberal ableism, the personal bodymind becomes the public basis on which to determine worth. For example, the increasing availability of genetic technologies—screening, diagnostic, and therapeutic tools—has coproduced what Kristin Bumiller refers to as a "conception of genetic normalcy," creating pressure (and means) for individuals to become personally responsible for genetic citizenship. She writes specifically on the geneticization of autism, which, despite having no definitive genetic marker, produces conditions under which pregnancies and children are scrutinized for their adherence to bodily and cognitive norms. Bumiller worries that this creates a "backdoor to eugenics," obscured by the rhetoric of personal autonomy that characterizes contemporary prenatal genetic testing. Genetic citizenship is less concerned with the reduction of suffering than with the optimization of health. Rather than having access to manage disease or disability as desired, individuals are expected to approximate an able-bodied/able-minded ideal. Driven by "the concurrent forces of life optimization . . . and demands for personal responsibility," genetic citizenship, as a manifestation of neoliberal ableism, judges a person's worthiness based on ability, genetic markers, and adherence to social norms.[29]

Neoliberal individual responsibility extends beyond the bodymind to any potential future bodyminds a person might produce. Scholars have paid particular attention to the pressure on prospective mothers, noting the explicitly gendered imbalance in accountability. In the context of prenatal genetic screening and diagnosis, which I explore in detail in the next chapter, with the dawn of routinized prenatal testing, women in effect "relinquished the right not to know."[30] Such responsibility comes into conflict with the rhetoric of autonomy and informed choice that undergirds contemporary American medicine. As Melinda Hall writes in her critique of transhumanist visions of a future in which there is "endless autonomy" but also a very narrow understanding of what constitutes an acceptable quality of life, "Parents must be responsible choosers, and so must their children."[31] The existence of technologies that enable us to *know,* that force choices where hitherto there were none, casts us, according to Ann Kerr and Tom Shakespeare, as increasingly "responsible for [our] own health and welfare."[32] Responsibility, in this case, almost universally means pursuing whatever knowledge—and intervention—modern medicine has made possible. To choose against knowledge acquisition and medical intervention is not only a personal moral failure but also a decision that jeopardizes the prosperity of the neoliberal market. Ironically, as the physical and cognitive abilities expected of an ideal citizen become ever more narrow, disability proliferates under neoliberalism.

This is not to suggest that individuals cannot or should not pursue medical care, or to invalidate individual experiences of pain, discomfort, or other elements of disability. Rather, it is to suggest that the reliance on medicine as a means of correcting or eliminating disability is intrinsically linked to political and social realities that produce and reproduce an idealized neoliberal subject.[33] This subject is perfectly independent, perfectly self-governing, and productive in a way that is legible and beneficial to the capitalist market. As such, as Michelle Murphy writes, "health seeking in the late twentieth century became a moral imperative that responsibilized individuals through risk."[34] Under this paradigm, a disabled bodymind is unruly, unworthy, and ungovernable unless the individual becomes self-responsible and pursues methods of body management such as those offered by medical technologies.

These conceptions of ableism underpin my analysis, extending beyond an abstract preference for ability by elucidating how this preference demands social, political, and ontological responsibility from individual actors. Coupled with the modern moral imperative to innovate, which confuses technological progress with social good, this neoliberal ableist paradigm paves the way for medicine as the de facto mode of intervention.[35]

Medicalization Matters

From sociology, I take insights about the cultural, historical, and ontological significance of medicalization. Medicalization, as understood by sociologist Peter Conrad, is the spread of medical jurisdiction into many aspects of human life. It is, most simply, the transformation of a human condition from a phenomenon outside medicine to one inside it. This process is largely definitional, as "a problem is defined in medical terms, described using medical language, understood through the adoption of a medical framework, or 'treated' with a medical intervention."[36] The subsuming of human experience into the powerful category of medicine serves to decontextualize and generalize personal and social conditions, in James Carrier's words, "misrecognizing and masking the effects of social practices and hierarchy."[37] For example, as congenital and developmental disabilities become increasing understood solely through genetic markers, the possibilities for intervention are constrained to only genetic diagnosis and termination before birth.[38]

The transformation of human phenomena into medical pathologies creates distinct social, political, ethical, and ontological relationships through the naming and standardization of fluid and contingent beings. As Peter Conrad and Joseph Schneider argue, medicalization's "greatest social power comes from having the authority to define certain behaviors, persons, and things."[39] Social control becomes legitimated through the pathologization of certain characteristics, aided by technologies that measure, quantify, and surveil the bodymind. Medicine's authority is so great that it declares what is ontologically, socially, and politically real.[40] Certain types of people and their knowledge become disavowed in this process, shifting into passive, receptive, and ultimately disposable roles.[41] The medicalization of disability specifically occludes the social arrangements that contribute to impairment. Geoffery Bowker and Susan Leigh Star have written extensively on the social and political power of medical classification; in their 1999 book *Sorting Things Out,* they feature this observation from 1958 as an epigraph: "How impracticable it is to try to classify human beings, for all time, into definite categories, and how much suffering has resulted from the efforts made to do this."[42] Medicalization forces fluid and evolving bodyminds and relationships into definitive and stable categories and freezes them there.

Disability emerges when social arrangements are incompatible with nonnormative bodyminds, rather than when a certain number of physiological characteristics are present simultaneously.[43] Technologies that provide biological data that can be interpreted as signifying disability, as well as those that intervene on biological characteristics, refute such claims and justify social systems that devalue and discriminate against disabled bodyminds. If disability is located within an individual's physiological systems, social institutions are not responsible for accommodating human variance. Rather, the individual is responsible for seeking treatment and management through medical intervention. The social conditions that cast disability as a medical problem contribute to and are informed by the construction and use of technologies that reinforce such thinking. Medical categorization invalidates other understandings of disability—for example, as a collective or individual identity—because "each standard and each category valorizes some point of view and silences another."[44] Situating a subject within a scientific purview may encourage the perception that the actions taken around it are objective. Kristina Gupta characterizes the distinct power dynamics of the professionalization of medicine, arguing that the medical establishment is itself stratified such that the people with the most authority to make decisions are those who already enjoy systemic privileges (by virtue of their race, gender, ability, and so on), which further alienates them from the experiences of many disabled people.[45] Thus, the principles and values that drive medical practice are often at odds with the desires and needs of disabled people.

Out of the expanding medicalization of life, the crush of technological innovation, and the proliferation of neoliberalism arose what medical sociologist Adele Clarke and colleagues refer to as "biomedicalization," or "the increasingly complex, multisited processes of medicalization that today are being both extended and reconstituted through the emergent social forms and practices of a highly and increasingly technoscientific biomedicine."[46] Pointing to the 1980s as the beginning of the biomedical era, they characterize biomedicalization as encompassing several unique processes, including the co-constitution of medical knowledge, technology, and capital; a focus on optimization and enhancement that authorizes surveillance; an increasing reliance on technoscience; transformations of knowledge and information systems; and the emergence of new technoscientific identities at both the individual and the collective level. These processes all bear critically on current experiences and expectations of medical technologies. As disability shifts to being understood primarily as biologically identifiable difference under a medical paradigm, it becomes decontextualized from its social and political vectors, which further reinforces the authority of medical experts to name and intervene on it.[47] Further, as medical authorities increasingly claim expertise, disabled people's experiences that are out of line with medical hegemony are frequently invalidated.

Challenges to user autonomy and responsible decision-making multiply as new technologies and procedures are developed, despite the fact that these values are at the core of Western medicine. The uncertainties of emerging technologies and procedures create contexts in which both the "informedness" and the "consentability" of informed consent come into question. "The lack of adequate information makes informed consent inconceivable," Mariachiara Tallacchini writes of xenotransplants, "and lays the basis for additional constraints to which patients have to consent."[48] She further suggests that new and experimental technologies expose their recipients not only to the burden of health risks but also to a lifetime of medical surveillance. Angela Willey and colleagues, writing about the social genealogy of autism, note a trend toward greater surveillance and control over nonnormative bodyminds.[49] On the other hand, Tiago Moreira and Paolo Palladino argue that informed consent and user autonomy become difficult to manage not because of surveillance and control but because of unreasonably high expectations due to exposure to a "regime of hope."[50] John Gardner, Gabrielle Samuel, and Clare Williams further assert that hope mobilizes innovation projects, even when visions of the future are "modest, uncertain, and ambivalent."[51] With hope comes obligation to act, because precluding hopeful futures seems morally unacceptable.

(Bio)medicalization is key to this research in that it makes explicit the contingencies through which disability is understood as a physiological or biological phenomenon. By elucidating the process of placing disability under medical jurisdiction, it opens up possibilities for understanding disability otherwise. The acknowledgment of medicalization reaffirms what the disability rights movement has asserted for many years: Disability is socially, politically, and materially constructed through human action. Medicine is as well.[52]

Technology Is Not Neutral

From feminist science and technology studies, I adopt the stance that the built world and technologies therein are neither neutrally constructed nor neutrally experienced. The technologies we use are embedded with the political and social values of the people who made them and their ideas about the people who use them—or the people on whom they are used.[53] In the context of medicine, this means that medical technologies do not exist to fill an a priori need. Instead, they play an active role in creating and perpetuating specific understandings of the bodymind. For example, as Ashley Shew writes of exoskeletons: "Existing narratives around paralysis (framed as an awful fate) and walking (assumed to be the best way of moving through the world) almost seem designed to end with exoskeletons as a solution to the 'problem' of mobility impairment—a technoableist's dream solution."[54] The design and use of medical technologies inform and are informed by social and cultural understandings of bodily and cognitive difference. Human experiences become standardized and reduced to a narrow set of clinically defined conditions in both the diagnostic and treatment processes. Technological intervention is valorized, which creates new pathways into both the physiological identification and individual treatment of disability, further cementing disability as a discretely biological phenomenon. Technologies enable a reduction and reclassification of people through standardization as a means of determining normality. People become compatible with the technologies used to quantify them.[55] This reduction, which quantifies messy human lives into orderly categories, is predicated on what can be measured and by what means. As John Gardner writes on deep brain stimulation, "The development and stabilisation of DBS therapies were contingent upon the co-development and diffusion of standardised methods of rendering the affected body."[56] The impacts of this standardization are manifold. New categories of people come into being through engagement with medical technology, with labels such as "at risk" allowing the boundaries of medical jurisdiction to creep ever outward.[57] Desires for measurable and actionable disease definitions lead to medical technologies that attribute mental and cognitive functioning to specific, detectable biological reactions.[58] The intensive, focused—and, as of this writing, unsuccessful—research devoted to identifying a single gene or set of genetic conditions that cause autism is one example of the increased pressure to attribute all human variation to discrete biological characteristics.

Further, reliance on quantification and direct observation in categorizing human variation tends to legitimate medical authority outside clinical spaces. The increasing entanglement of social classifications with medical classifications has impacts on disabled people regardless of their individual engagement with health care and medical technology. Individual biological and physiological characteristics are bundled together and gain legal, political, and social significance, such as through diagnostic requirements for access to social services. At the same time, medical authorities claim sole credibility to identify syndromes, disabilities, and chronic illness, thus intensifying the social construction of disability as medical pathology.

Technology can and does play an active role in this process. In discussing the concept of the social construction of technology, Trevor Pinch and Wiebe Bijker suggest that the "sociocultural and political situation of a social group shapes its norms and values, which in turn influence the meaning given to [a technology]."[59] Their symmetrical approach circumvents normative assumptions about what should or should not be and instead examines how certain technologies come to be favored over others. This is a particularly useful way of looking at technologies associated with disability. Rather than assuming that diagnostic and intervention technologies are developed to fill obvious needs in identifying and eliminating disability, I can instead explore the reciprocal relationship between medical technologies and the social and political structures that insist on disability as undesirable. For example, diagnostic tools like prenatal genetic testing contribute to framing disability as both detectable and manageable through medical intervention. At the same time, the social conditions that pathologize disability as in need of elimination contribute to the development and use of these technologies. As Ilana Löwy writes of prenatal genetic testing, "The complex nexus of the relationship between academic science and private industry . . . made possible the incorporation of ideals of individual choice, risk management and responsible parenthood into circulating, marketable items."[60] In a social context that privileges a physiological explanation for disability and insists on individual responsibility, diagnostic technologies are favored over technologies that address socioeconomic disparities. The existence of a medical technology reifies its target as something in need of intervention as well as the correct mechanism through which to intervene.

Following from the above insights, the distinctions between material reality and social worlds blur. It is not simply that one informs the other, but that they are co-constituted and mutually reinforcing. Drawing rigid distinctions between nature and culture—and then announcing sovereignty over one or the other—is simultaneously the hallmark of modernity and a paradoxical impossibility, according to Bruno Latour.[61] He opts instead for attention to the hybridization, the "nature-cultures" and networks in which humans and nonhumans act and interact, and in which knowledge, belief, and science hold equal epistemological weight. Toward my purposes, this approach unsettles taken-for-granted distinctions between the natural (biological or physiological) and the social (differential values ascribed to certain bodily arrangements) in thinking about disability. Further, it rejects the idea that a natural "truth" can and must be uncovered through the application of the right set of methods and knowledges. Disability, then, is not something that materially exists waiting to be identified, nor is it solely a social or political phenomenon; rather, as feminist science and technology studies scholar Karen Barad writes, "the material and the discursive are mutually implicated."[62] As explored above, to understand disability under this paradigm is to recognize it as infinitely contingent; there is no set of biological or physiological symptoms that definitively signal disability. Rather, the social and material dimensions of disability are co-constituted as a means of producing and maintaining order. Barad's "posthumanist account" extends attention to the entanglement of the social and the material by "call[ing] into question the givenness of the differential categories . . . [and] examining the practices through which these differential boundaries are stabilized and destabilized."[63] Such work becomes particularly useful when it is applied to an analysis of medical technologies that are designed and deployed in a context in which the "givenness" of disability as both materially real and socially undesirable is assumed.

Embodiment and Experience Are Legitimate Sources of Knowledge

I am concerned with questions of authority and legitimacy to define disability and mandate appropriate responses, questions that at their core deal with how knowledge is produced. Knowledge, however, is not simply a statement of truth but also a dynamically constructed, fluid process. The social, political, and material conditions that privilege one type of knowledge claim subjugate other ways of knowing and being. Therefore, out of feminist epistemologies, I carry into this analysis the assumption that knowledge produced through embodiment and experience is both valid and underutilized in medical settings. Like scholars of science and technology studies, feminist epistemologies reject the notion of an objective or neutral framework as the only allowable path to truth. According to feminist scholar Sandra Harding, adherence to positivist frameworks does not cultivate neutrality; on the contrary, it perpetuates and obscures bias.[64] By rejecting positivism, we make space to consider situated knowledges: contingent, partial, and subjective knowledges that arise from the unique social position each individual occupies.[65] I take for granted the validity of experiential and embodied knowledge claims. Drawing from science studies literature, Harding argues that science, despite its veneer of neutrality, is intrinsically shaped by the politics of "dominant institutions, structures, priorities, research strategies, technologies, and languages of the sciences."[66] This facade of objectivity cements an authoritarian science. Sexism, racism, colonialism, classism, and ableism are baked into the traditional scientific endeavor, but they are depoliticized through claims of detachment. Harding writes that "in hierarchically organized societies, the daily activities of the ruling groups tend to set distinctive limits on their thought, limits that are not created by the activities of subjugated groups"; more saliently, she points out that the work of the natural and social sciences is a form of ruling in contemporary societies.[67] Similar to other feminist scholars invested in knowledge production, Harding ultimately argues that recognizing positionality allows for the generation of more authentic truth claims than can come from a supposedly neutral scientific approach that does not acknowledge the social, political, and individual contexts in which individuals are enmeshed.[68] Such an insight is in line with Pinch and Bijker's sociological examination of scientific knowledge; they assert that "there is nothing epistemologically special about the nature of scientific knowledge. It is merely one in a whole series of knowledge cultures."[69] Further, interrogating the perspectives, knowledge practices, and expertise of users, patients, and other stakeholders with limited power is imperative for understanding the nature of agency and accountability under a medicalized regime. As Bowker and Star note, "If social scientists do not understand people's definition of a situation, they do not understand it at all."[70]

Second, and relatedly, as in the lineage of feminist disability studies, I take for granted that the misfit between disabled bodyminds and a material-discursive world that was constructed for and by nondisabled people produces contexts in which disabled people have unique knowledge about that world. Rosemarie Garland-Thomson argues that misfitting is contingent and particular—there is no generic disabled bodymind that could dematerialize in the right environment. She also suggests that misfitting confers agency and value by emphasizing resourcefulness, adaptability, and knowledge. Importantly, a misfit is not the result of an inherent wrongness in either the bodymind or the environment; rather, it arises from their spatial and temporal juxtaposition. Disability, then, is a "way of being in an environment, a material arrangement."[71] Disability and science studies scholars have suggested, both directly and indirectly, that the positionality of disabled, ill, or otherwise medically subjugated bodyminds allows them access to knowledge not available to others. Tobin Siebers calls out the value of a disabled standpoint in presenting his disability theory, stating that he is motivated by "the contention that oppressed social locations create identities and perspectives, embodiments and feelings, histories and experiences that stand outside of and offer valuable knowledge about the powerful ideologies that seem to enclose us." He continues: "While all identities contain social knowledge, mainstream identities are less critical . . . because they are normative. Minority identities acquire the ability to make epistemological claims about the society in which they hold liminal positions, owing precisely to their liminality."[72]

In the chapters that follow, I privilege the accounts of disabled people in both my case analyses and my ultimate recommendations. In the case of deep brain stimulation and DIY diabetes technologies, the majority of informants I spoke with identified as disabled or chronically ill. In the case of prenatal genetic screening and testing, however, the majority of informants did not identify as disabled. During those interviews, I was instead attentive to the notable *absence* of disabled embodiment in discussions of congenital difference. Taking seriously embodiment as a source of knowledge, I trouble the demarcation of scientific knowledge as exceptional, instead forcing an examination of the social positions that animate all knowledge claims. Such an approach ameliorates the tension between disabled and nondisabled, recognizing both as contingent and subsequently valuing what emerges from the mismatch. Difference becomes relational, not essential. Further, misfitting becomes an epistemic resource that produces generative possibilities for alternative ways of knowing and being.

Through this chapter, I have articulated an epistemological context for medical technologies that detect, intervene on, or eliminate disability. The slipperiness of disability as a category lends particular social and political power to medical technologies that, by their existence, mark their targets for intervention as both ontologically real and undesirable. Set against the backdrop of neoliberal ableism and (bio)medicalization, the development, use, and narratives of medical technologies challenge and reject alternative epistemologies, particularly those rooted in lived experience. I argue, however, that such epistemologies yield critical knowledge about a material-discursive world constructed on curative logics. The schema outlined in this chapter structures my interpretation of the three case studies that follow. I now turn to the first of these cases to demonstrate the entanglement of knowledge and responsibility in prenatal genetic screening and testing.

« 2 »

Becoming Responsible with Prenatal Genetic Testing

When she found out she was expecting her first child, Melanie, an academic professional living in the Southwest United States, freely admitted that she knew next to nothing about pregnancy. At her first appointment with her midwife, she told me, "they do a full pelvic exam, and then they get very, very personal." While she was in the stirrups, Melanie recalled, the clinician asked about her and her partner's familial histories, and "it doesn't go well, let's just say that." Heritable and genetic conditions, gaps in their knowledge due to adoption and missing paperwork, and their ethnic backgrounds all meant that Melanie and her partner were immediately referred to a genetic counselor. Melanie spoke of the deflating feeling of receiving that referral just minutes after having her pregnancy confirmed:

> We didn't really get to celebrate because all of a sudden all these questions got brought to us, you know, whatever. So, then [comes] the conversation about a [genetic] counselor and I'm like, "Well I don't even know what this is. Like, what does this mean? What do we do?"

Upon meeting with her genetic counselor, Melanie was immediately confronted with a choice: Given her history, what kind of genetic screening did she want to pursue? She was offered several options, but she never felt that she had the choice of not doing the screening. "It sounds very scary," she said, of learning about her personal risk factors. "And I'm a rational person, a logical person, so I thought I shouldn't be as nervous, but I think it's the way that they present everything that you start to like, 'Well what if I don't do this?' And then whatever happens." As she was sorting through screening options, the counselor warned her against pursuing a full genetic panel, which would test for many more genetic markers than the typical screening offers:

> And [the genetic counselor] goes, "Be careful with that one," which I was very happy that she gave some type of like idea about it, because who wouldn't want to know everything, right? If you had the opportunity to know everything about your genetic background and your baby's genetic background, like, do it. But then she did warn, like, "You do that you're going to find something." . . . We knew right away that we weren't going to do the full panel one because both of us would have gone nuts.

At the same time, Melanie was experiencing health complications, including debilitating morning sickness that led to hospitalization. She recalled the strain of this time period. She and her partner were not particularly concerned with having a child with a disability, just with carrying the pregnancy to term: "It was a lot of me randomly crying," she said. "Not only because of my hormones, but because, like, I was so scared to lose our son. Because all this [genetic screening] didn't tell me whether that meant I'm more at risk to lose a child or not. Like, none of that told me."

This chapter juxtaposes interviews with prospective parents like Melanie, interviews with genetic counselors and clinicians, and user-directed materials produced by hospitals and commercial genetic screening companies to interrogate the relationships among prenatal genetic screening and diagnosis, knowledge accumulation as an obligation of responsible parenting, and the construction of congenital disability.[1] In the prenatal clinic, the meaning of "disability" is multiple. Clinicians favor biological, visualizable constructions, locating disability discretely in extra chromosomes or translocated segments. Both professionals and parents, however, acknowledge social, educational, and relational dimensions of disability as important information for making decisions about pregnancy management. But this knowledge remains slippery and uncertain, particularly in the absence of disabled embodied knowledge in the clinic. Further, clinical constructions of disability figure it as either a tragedy or an inspiration, two perspectives that are equally dehumanizing. The privileging of the physiological conditions of disability at the expense of sharing knowledge about social and political realities ultimately undermines the rhetoric of autonomy and informed consent that undergirds PGT and genetic counseling. Further, prospective parents express frustration at this partial knowledge and are often forced to rely on external sources such as online forums and parent support groups. This exposes the limitations of medical professionals' assumptions about what information is most salient during pregnancy management. Ultimately, I expose the perceived obligatory nature of screening and testing in pursuit of responsible parenthood—particularly a gendered and classed responsible motherhood—and tensions between the knowledge sought by prospective parents and that proffered by professionals. I end by arguing that PGT simultaneously materializes disability through genetic material and disembodies it by abstracting the future disabled child entirely, leaving little room for embodied and experiential knowledge in technology development and clinical interactions.

Genetic (Un)certainty

In April 2022, the U.S. Food and Drug Administration released a warning regarding the validity and use of noninvasive prenatal screening. This screening method, which analyzes fetal or placental DNA circulating in a pregnant person's bloodstream, has exploded in popularity since it became commercially available in the United States in the early 2010s.[2] Requiring only a blood draw, in contrast to the riskier and more invasive procedures used in other diagnostic testing, such as amniocentesis, NIPS is appealing in its simplicity, safety, and possible use early in pregnancy. NIPS predicts the likelihood of a broad scope of fetal conditions, from common ones caused by aneuploidies (too many or too few copies of chromosomes), like Down syndrome, to extremely rare, sometimes singular, conditions caused by the deletion or duplication of small sections of chromosomes. However, as the FDA warns, "many laboratories offering [NIPS] advertise their tests as 'reliable' and 'highly accurate,' offering 'peace of mind' for patients. The FDA is concerned that that these claims may not be supported with sound scientific evidence."[3] In 2019, the UK-based Nuffield Council on Bioethics published a blog sharing similar concerns, stating that NIPS results in very high false positive rates, even for common aneuploidies. For example, it noted a 60 percent false positive rate for

Edwards syndrome, caused by an extra copy of chromosome 18. In addition to these uncertain outcomes, the Nuffield Council warned about poor-quality information about the conditions screened for and lack of follow-up support for prospective parents.[4]

Despite such misgivings, NIPS is becoming standardized in pregnancy management. In 2019, molecular biologist Dennis Lo Yuk-ming, a key figure in the development of NIPS, stated that more than six million women across ninety countries had received such screening.[5] NIPS is intended to serve as a first-level screening, with the assumption that users will pursue more invasive diagnostic testing to confirm any positive results as their pregnancies progress. However, with increasing restrictions on access to abortion in the United States owing to the overturning of *Roe v. Wade* in the summer of 2022, the window to terminate a pregnancy following prenatal screening has closed for many. For those living in states that have gestational limits, further diagnostic testing may not be possible. Amniocentesis, for example, is typically done between weeks 14 and 20, with increased risk of complications if it is done earlier.[6] Therefore, the uncertain, but convincingly packaged, knowledge produced by NIPS may be the only information available to people who need to make pregnancy management decisions.

Pregnant people and their partners, then, are stuck in a bind. They are expected to seek out as much knowledge as possible about their pregnancies in order to act as rational and responsible parents. As one commercial lab's website reads, "Knowing the relevant genetic information about your pregnancy is one of the first steps in planning for a happy and healthy family." At the same time, the tools prospective parents have at their disposal for seeking out that knowledge are not always reliable, although their use is couched in a rhetoric of accuracy, certainty, and scientific credibility. Further, the information deemed relevant in pregnancy management decision-making rarely, if ever, includes information gained from the lived experiences of disabled people.

Knowing and Not Knowing

Melanie's anecdote presented at the opening of this chapter exemplifies how genetic knowledge can be constructed as a means of empowerment or as a source of unnecessary anxiety. In almost all of the interviews, informants explained or justified PGT as a way of accumulating essential knowledge for responsible pregnancy management. But prospective parents and professionals also drew a distinction between "necessary" knowledge and knowledge that would only result in undue stress. How they delineated those categories, however, was left tacit. A lack of explicit articulation of why some conditions demanded testing while others did not reinforces the idea that disability is easily definable and obviously requires identification and intervention. Additionally, prospective parents felt as if there were significant gaps in their knowledge, a suspicion bolstered by professionals' confirmation that they presented certain knowledge based on assumptions made about prospective parents. These knowledge gaps were exacerbated by the inherent uncertainty of PGT itself. This section highlights a distinct set of knowledge expectations and practices that characterize the experience of prenatal genetic testing and screening. These practices are largely inferred and ill-defined, leading to dissatisfaction and anxiety among prospective parents.

A "Nice Foundation of Evidence": Empowerment and Anxiety in Knowledge Accumulation

Almost universally across the interviews, informants suggested that PGT provides some essential knowledge that empowers prospective parents to make informed decisions about pregnancy management. Gene, an academic professional whose partner received PGT in both of her pregnancies, suggested that he and his partner pursued testing because their professional background as researchers predisposed them to gather and analyze as many data as possible when making decisions. He told me, "We were both social scientists. We like some kind of nice foundation of evidence to at least provide a sense of security or comfort, if nothing else."

Often, such language of empowerment was used specifically during discussions of scenarios in which an abnormal testing result would not lead to termination of the pregnancy. Abby, who strongly opposed abortion for religious reasons, initially balked at the idea of PGT, linking it in her mind only to termination. Eventually, however, the allure of knowledge, which she decided could assist her and her partner in making decisions around care, drew her to the idea of receiving NIPS. She said:

> So, then we were like, "We're not going to do it, because it doesn't matter, because we're going to keep the baby. It's irrelevant." But then, we're like, "Well, we kind of want to know because if there is something, it's not going to affect the outcome, but it would affect all of our care up to that point," because then we would want to see specialists. We would want to maybe deliver at [a large medical research center] instead of at [the local hospital] if there's going to be an issue. We'd want to have specialists lined up.

She eventually conceded that curiosity convinced them to pursue screening, telling me, "Honestly, just wanting to know is kind of the bottom line, is because we didn't know and it's something that you could know so easily and then decide, 'Okay, what are we going to do for it?' So just wanting to know, the curiosity of it." She continued by suggesting that the knowledge NIPS can provide about gender served as extra protection against potential backlash from others who associate PGT with pregnancy termination: "We'll just say we want to do it for the gender and then it won't look bad."

The ease of knowledge acquisition and almost nonexistent health risk to the fetus or pregnant person influenced other prospective parents to pursue noninvasive screening technologies as well. Rosalie, who was pregnant at the time of her interview, stated, "Since it's not an [amniocentesis] anymore, since it's something you can test without a risk of miscarriage, I'm all for making really informed decisions. So, I was all about it." Theresa, a genetic counselor, confirmed that noninvasive testing appeals to risk-averse prospective parents, noting:

> I think that a less invasive test is more powerful for those types of patients. Because these are the ones who are more likely to have testing now because they're like, "You know what? I kind of would like to know ahead of time. I would never have an amnio, but if I am at risk for having a baby with Down syndrome, I would want to know in advance. I would want to prepare, I would want to maybe, you know, deliver elsewhere."

Here again, testing was associated with preparedness for a future disabled child rather than with pregnancy termination.

This framing of testing as frictionless knowledge empowerment obscures the tensions and anxieties experienced by prospective parents. While both prospective parents and professionals discussed knowledge accumulation as a form of empowerment, informants who were prospective parents were much more likely to see it as a potential source of anxiety as well. When making this point, however, they were clear to distinguish between an "appropriate" level of knowledge, which often was synonymous with whatever suite of testing was recommended by their clinician, and "too much" knowledge, which often included things like full genomic workups or advanced testing options, as exemplified by Melanie's anecdote above. Patsy noted that she would rather have had the option of no testing, but as someone receiving fertility treatments, she did not feel as though she could decline. "But I kind of would rather take it hands-off," she said. "You know, as long as whatever's healthy for me. I kind of would rather leave it like 'It is what it is.'" The rhetoric of optionality is even less present in fertility clinics than in prenatal settings, as nearly all fertility clinics require screening of embryos prior to implantation. Patsy's discomfort, like Melanie's, stemmed from the possibility of knowing too much, which in her case would force her into a position to make decisions about what kind of child she would like to bring into the world, a situation that she noted she did not see occurring in nonassisted pregnancies. Through testing, she would become responsible for new kinds of decisions that otherwise would not have been possible.

The majority of analyzed user-directed documents, regardless of source, suggested that PGT provides knowledge that empowers prospective parents to make decisions, resonating with the experiences of both interviewed prospective parents and medical professionals. Specifically, PGT was presented as creating opportunities for informed decision-making, eliding the fact that it also creates new sets of choices that otherwise would not need to be made. One professional society, for example, lists "empowerment" among the reasons people opt for genetic testing writ large. Commercial genetic testing companies pepper their websites and brochures with affirmations about the power of knowledge, using taglines such as "Before hello, it helps to know," "The confidence you seek, with fewer risks," and "Parents who know can make steps to prepare." All of the resources strongly emphasized that prospective parents should make decisions in concert with or at the recommendation of experts and professionals, however, suggesting that laypersons need assistance in identifying what knowledge is appropriate for them. Very few addressed the anxiety of knowing "too much." One professional society did allude to knowledge anxiety, noting, "Some may choose not to get tested because they find the risk of getting a positive result too stressful, especially in cases when there is no treatment available." However, there was very little in the documentation, especially from commercial companies, offering prospective parents any help in sorting through their options. Instead, it was implied that most decisions around what testing and screening to pursue would be made on their behalf in the clinic.

"Do You Want to Continue or Do You Want to Terminate?": Knowledge Conflicts in the Clinic

Prospective parent informants spoke to a number of common experiences around how clinicians delivered information and what information they delivered. Overwhelmingly, prospective parents felt inadequately informed. This applied to testing and screening as well as to pregnancy more broadly. By way of response, many medical professionals I spoke to revealed how and when they decide to share information with prospective parents, with their decisions often based on assumptions about both the prospective parents in question and the broader social system in which they are embedded. For example, genetic counselor Julia noted that she shares information about adoption only when the prenatal diagnosis is Down syndrome, as she is personally familiar with an adoption agency that specializes in this. "For anything else," she said, "It's going to be 'Do you want to continue, or do you want to terminate?'"

Abby noted that she had a particularly difficult time getting her clinician to discuss potential next steps with her prior to receiving her testing results, and that made her feel underprepared to make decisions when the results did come in. She shared:

> I'm always like, okay, worst-case scenario, what happens? And I need to have that idea in my head of, okay, what's going to happen if A, then what? Or if B, then what? That's something that I would've liked to know, what's going to happen if I get a positive result?

She supplemented the limited information she got from her clinician with independent research at home, which made her feel more capable of making decisions.

Genetic counselor Julia also acknowledged prospective parents' desire for more knowledge, particularly knowledge linked to lived experience:

> I think, you know, overall, the impression I get from patients is what they wanna hear is, you know, might the child be able to live and work on their own one day? Is the child going to need help long-term? Or is the child not going to make it out of infancy?

For prospective parents like Melanie and Patsy, it was not *what* information was shared but *how* it was shared that made an impression. Melanie, as described above, was understandably overwhelmed when her clinician began asking about her familial history of genetic conditions while conducting a pelvic exam at her first appointment. Patsy received the results of her carrier testing in a PDF that was blazoned with misleading labels like "Positive" and "Negative" while what were actually being described were probabilities. Patsy has a background in genetics that enabled her to navigate the report, but she noted that she worried for others: "I would kind of feel for someone else who got these PDFs that was looking through them and wasn't really sure what 'positive' means and what that means for their health." She added, "It's probably scary."

In the interviews, both prospective parents and professionals noted that misconceptions about the testing process itself could produce stress. Several prospective parents, like Melanie, felt pressure and anxiety when initially presented with the recommendation to visit a genetic counselor and receive a screening test, as they had little understanding of what that meant. Genetic counselor Miriam noted that many prospective parents come to see her without knowing what genetic screening is. "Some will say, 'Oh, well my OB just said it was an option, so here I am,'" she recounted, "and some are like, 'I really don't know what I'm here for.'" She and the majority of the other medical professionals interviewed suggested that, given the wide range of knowledge and experience they encounter, one of their primary roles is that of information provider.

While Patsy's and Abby's concerns described above both arose from inadequate interactions with their medical providers, Marcie's stemmed from professional overinvolvement. Marcie has been a practicing genetic counselor for forty years and had also served as director of a genetic counseling master's program, and so has spent much time reflecting on the tensions between training and practice. She suggested that in the clinical setting, the genetic counselor's aspiration to "nondirectiveness," as emphasized in training, guidance documents, and informational documents for prospective parents, is not really achievable. She emphasized the cognitive dissonance between training and the human reality of practice:

> You know, you can never—we do this sort of nonsense of "be a nondirective counselor," yeah, yeah, yeah, you know? [laughs] And we strive for that, and it's good to do that, but yes there's a piece of yourself that has to go into this, otherwise, you're a robot.

This statement is in tension with prospective parents' tendency to view clinicians as neutral producers of salient information. As Marcie made clear, the human element of clinical work inherently shifts what and how information is communicated, in a way that prospective parents may not be privy to.

"We Can't Predict What's Going to Happen to Your Child": Uncertainty

Uncertainty characterized many informants' experiences of PGT. Some, like Gene, framed PGT as mitigating some uncertainties, a valuable benefit, given the inherent uncertainty of raising a child. "We know there is going to be a whole host of curveballs and surprises of every different kind, of different scales," Gene told me, "so, some of it we'll have a clue of what to expect and others we won't." Abby, on the other hand, resented the certainty with which PGT was presented to her and her partner, feeling that their clinician represented the testing as providing a definitive statement of fetal health:

> It's definitely presented as this is the genetic testing and if you pass, then you're going to have an okay baby. And never mind the billions of other things that could go astray during the DNA sequencing process. No, only three things ever go wrong with that, okay.

Abby's irritation at this misrepresentation of PGT was echoed in many of the interviews conducted with genetic counselors, several of whom expressed concerns that other medical professionals, including obstetricians and office staff, misunderstand the testing and pass their own false certainty on to users. Theresa, who works as a medical liaison for a commercial PGT company, suggested that the misconceptions that arise among clinicians come in part from "a little bit of heightened excitement and a little bit of, you know, that allure and that sexiness of DNA testing in general," and this leads to the perpetuation of misinformation in clinics. Sabrina, a geneticist, and Marcie both argued that genetics should be featured more prominently in medical school curricula. They noted that knowledge about genetics has become especially crucial given the increased routinization of genetic testing, as more and more prospective parents now receive testing without ever interacting with genetic counselors. Several professionals also noted a need for increased awareness and education among others in medical and professional positions, especially clinic staff.

As Marcie said when I inquired about prospective parents' (mis)understandings about screening and testing, "We can't predict what's going to happen to your child, we can't predict for any child." She and other interviewed professionals consistently reinforced the uncertainty of testing and screening, and were adamant about their efforts to resist and rebuff the misconceptions they encounter. It is notable that both prospective parents and professionals claimed awareness of the uncertainty of PGT, implicitly constructing a third category of misinformed or uninformed users. Some professionals, like geneticist Sabrina and genetic counselor Julia, felt that misconceptions are being perpetuated or exacerbated by commercial entities that produce genetic tests. Julia said that she is not always able to address misunderstandings because of the involvement of private companies: "Some of [the misconceptions are] because it's not in our hands, it's in the hands of the privates, and they just say, 'Oh, everything's fine, it's perfect, you don't have to worry about anything.'"

Sabrina, who has been a researcher in genetic screening and therapy for many years, also attributed many of the misunderstandings about PGT to the speed of rollout by commercial companies and misleading marketing. Of NIPS specifically, she said:

> Part of the problem, but part of the opportunity, was that the initial testing and the rollout of the testing was done by industry. Things would never have happened as fast as they did without the capacity of industry. But in retrospect, some of the marketing associated with the testing, particularly beginning when some of the companies said, "This is as good as an amniocentesis," led to the confusion that this was a diagnostic test. We've been trying to walk that back for many years now to say it's a screening test.

Uncertainty featured heavily in nearly all analyzed documentation. Often, this was in the form of liability statements from commercial companies. The phrase "No test is perfect" appeared verbatim on two commercial sites and one health system informational page, while others emphasized that screening and testing do not promise the "perfect" child. One reminded prospective parents that "even when all the results of diagnostic testing are normal, all pregnancies still have approximately a 3–5% risk of birth defects." A professional society highlighted uncertainty even further, emphasizing that genetics are not the only factor relevant in a fetus's health and development, stating, "It's also important to understand that genes don't determine everything."

Most guidance documents emphasized the need for professional guidance or intervention in the use of PGT. As one hospital system stated, "Talking to your doctor, a medical geneticist or a genetic counselor about what you will do with the results is an important step in the process of genetic testing." Expert guidance, in this case, could also be read as gatekeeping: access to certain kinds of knowledge, including some types of screening or testing and genetic counseling, is possible only "*at your physician's direction*" (emphasis added). The appearance of this gatekeeping in the documentation reaffirmed the experiences of the prospective parents, who felt inadequately informed about the screening and testing process. In terms of understanding and misunderstanding the technology itself, only a third of the documents provided any detail on the processes and science behind PGT (and usually only in the context of noninvasive prenatal testing). Again, the importance of a clinical expert or guide was emphasized, with a professional society stating, "Many couples do not realize what these tests may or may not tell them, so meeting with a genetic counselor prior to having cfDNA [cell-free DNA] or other prenatal screening tests is highly recommended."

Despite this recommendation, most pregnant people cannot access genetic counselors, and instead rely on other clinicians or commercial entities for knowledge. Overall, the documentation supported the interpretation of PGT as a provider of knowledge that serves to empower prospective parents, as long as it is delivered under the watchful eye of the clinicians they encounter.

Constructing Disability

As part of her job as a genetic counselor, Julia is often the one responsible for explaining the results of a prenatal genetic screening or diagnostic test. This means she may be the first person ever to present information about disability to a prospective family. In speaking with her, it became clear that this is a responsibility she takes seriously. She told me:

> Some of the feedback I get as well, particularly with Down syndrome is, "It was all doom and gloom, and nobody told me how wonderful it could be to raise a child that has Down syndrome." And while I am empathetic to that, my professional opinion is if I don't tell you the worst of it, I have not done my job, and from a litigation perspective, it would be particularly dangerous for me. So, I try not to be all doom and gloom, I try to be balanced, but it is my personal and professional opinion that we've got to get some of the bad news out there in addition to some of the, you know, "Families can be happy with kids with this condition stuff out there as well."

Julia's statement sums up the complexities of constructing disability within the prenatal genetic testing apparatus. In this section, I explore the nuanced and conflicting ways in which disability comes to be understood by clinicians and prospective parents, which in turn frames decisions around pregnancy management. Often, mirroring broader social constructions, disability is established along two binaries. Most of the professionals interviewed made a stark distinction between the medical and social dimensions of disability, with the majority relying heavily on physiological and medicalized frameworks. Both parents and medical professionals discussed disabled children in two specific and contrasting tenors: as tragedies or as valuable or inspirational lessons for nondisabled parents and societies. Additionally, the uncertainty of the presence or absence of disability, alongside the presence and absence of the fetus during pregnancy, creates a sense of liminality: For some, pregnancy becomes "real" only after testing is complete. For others, making pregnancy management decisions is possible because the fetus is, to quote prospective parent Abby, "not a person yet."

This theme raises important questions about the framing of disability in clinical contexts, linking it in important ways to questions of knowledge production, autonomy, and authority. Prospective parents' access to knowledge—and therefore their ability to make informed decisions—is constrained by the categorical framing of congenital disability. As Anton, a prenatal and preconception genetic counselor in the Great Plains region, questioned when discussing whether to bring fetuses with life-threatening genetic conditions to term or to perform therapeutic treatments on such newborns, "Well, a lot of people would say no, we shouldn't do that because these babies don't have a real high quality of life, but then who decides what's the quality of life?"

"This Is Very Tangible": Emphasizing Pathology in the Clinic

Both prospective parents and medical professionals made a distinction between medical information about disability, such as risk or presence of physiological differences, and social information about disability, such as a future child's potential to learn, develop, and live independently. Despite a variety of experiences with disabled people both within and outside the clinic, genetic counselors showed some similarities in how they understood and interpreted disability in counseling sessions. The majority of genetic counselors interviewed either explicitly stated or implicitly suggested that the conceptualizations of disability they presented to their patients strongly favored biological characteristics. Miriam, who had been working as a genetic counselor for a little over a year at the time of our interview, flatly stated, "Um, I'm trying to—honestly, I will say I focus more on the medical side of it." Others shared Julia's perspective above, reporting a perceived obligation to communicate worst-case scenarios resulting from genetic diagnosis.

Anton suggested that biological probabilities, even if not yet manifested in the fetus, are more predictable and less complex than social outcomes or even phenotypic presentations. When speaking about 22q deletion, a genetic condition associated with schizophrenia, he said:

> The hard thing is like, social context. It may [be] your baby's going to get a heart defect because this is a very tangible— this is the next thing; you do heart surgery. Versus, they might develop a mental health issue, schizophrenia, at some point, that's—then you're like on pins and needles, like, are they gonna get this, and when are they gonna get that? That's a lot harder to discuss prenatally because it's not tangible, there's not a next step, it's kind of a wait-and-see and hope that it doesn't happen type of thing.

Perceptions of disability held by genetic counselors were informed by their experiences with disabled people.[7] Often, these interactions were in short-term, highly structured settings, such as a rotation in a day service program during training, or in a medicalized environment, such as a general genetics clinic. These settings overwhelmingly constructed disability as pathology. Carmen, who works as a prenatal genetic counselor in an office that provides first-trimester screenings, recalled a rotation in her training in which she was surprised to encounter adults with congenital conditions resulting in significant disabilities, noting that she "wouldn't have ever expected to see someone alive with that condition."

Julia remarked that her most substantial experience with disability occurred in a clinical setting. She recounted the time immediately following her training nearly forty years prior, describing it as frightening. She shared the story with an air of morbid fascination:

> When I started, I started in general genetics, and the geneticist that I worked for said, "Consider this your internship here."

> And I really felt—I walked around with a little notebook, and I wrote down all the terms I didn't understand, even though I had done the medical genetics course, and we did medical terminology, when you see a kid with Down syndrome, you never forget it. I can remember we had a kid with microcephaly, and we had some random deletion, and he had status epilepticus and needed to be admitted. And I don't think I'd worked there three months. And my boss hands him to me, stiff as a board because he's seizing so much, and says, "Help [the child's mother] to admissions, and go up to the floor with her." And I'm holding this kid, who's probably nine or ten years old, three feet long, seizing away. I was terrified. That's how you learn.

Such limited and clinical exposures to disability inform personal meanings, which in turn seep into professional exchanges.

"The Devastation It Can Wreak on Households": Disability as Tragedy or Inspiration

The second binary that emerged was one that constructed disability as either a personal tragedy or an inspiration, lesson, or gift to a nondisabled community. The former rendering of disability was often found in negatively connotative language rather than outright statements. For example, Rosalie, when discussing her worries about her testing results, said, "There is a definite before and after to me . . . because of the anxieties I had around all that kind of high-risk, horrible stuff." Gene, a prospective parent, described feeling grateful upon learning that the screening did not raise any concerns about genetic conditions, admitting, "The devastation it can wreak on households and oh I can't even . . . financial, emotional, I can't even fathom some of this." Counselor Carmen, when discussing disability with prospective patients, noted, "I try obviously to be gentle with it [laughs], you know, when I'm talking the social aspects of it because they can be, depending on the condition, very devastating." Miriam shared that while she often encounters prospective parents with positive understandings of genetic conditions, especially Down syndrome, she feels it necessary to reorient them to recognize the potential negative outcomes:

> And I will say, "Yeah, I'm glad to hear you had some pleasant interactions with people with Down syndrome, there are

definitely lots of people with Down syndrome out there who have a great life. They are able to do these jobs that you see them doing, and I'm—they're smiling and whatnot." And I say, "But unfortunately that is not the case for everybody."

Other professionals, like Marcie, who works as both a genetic counselor and an educator, recognized that historically, medical professionals have been complicit in constructing a universally negative picture of disability. She noted recent adjustments to training and practice, particularly in the rhetoric used to discuss disability. For example, she shared that she personally no longer offers condolences when offering a genetic diagnosis:

I used to. I used to. And it—I would say it was culturally appropriate then. It's no longer appropriate. So, we don't. We don't say that anymore. We sometimes say, "I'm sorry your test result didn't turn out the way you wanted," because that is. But not, "I'm sorry your baby has Down syndrome."

However, even the modified statement Marcie mentioned assumes prospective parents' investment in nondisabledness. The conscious recognition of how discourse shapes perceptions was not singular to Marcie's interview but was not found in the majority of interviews.

Additionally, despite their pivotal role in identifying, explaining, and, in some cases, assisting in the management of pregnancies involving disability, counselors relayed complex and varied orientations and engagements with existing disability communities. Often, they highlighted tensions, as these communities can act simultaneously as resources for prospective parents and as vocal critics of genetic counseling and prenatal genetic testing as a practice. The majority of the professionals stated that they regularly refer prospective parents to these communities (in an informal manner that cannot be verified or followed up on), but four counselors also cited oppositional relationships to some disability communities. Julia expressed the feeling that her profession is misunderstood, noting that there is "animosity in feeling like there's seek-and-destroy." All interviewed counselors refuted the criticisms raised by disability communities, arguing that counselors serve as patient advocates. This real or perceived hostility, however, may dissuade professionals from referring prospective parents to disability communities, and thus risks further essentializing disability to its biological components by alienating crucial embodied and experiential experts such as disabled people and their families.

On the opposite end of this constructed binary is the perception that disability is a valuable addition to a community. As Theresa shared, when she encountered people resistant to genetic counseling because of its potentially eugenic applications, she framed the conversation this way:

> [Make] sure that people are on the same page about, right, children with Down syndrome are enriching, they enrich our lives, and they are beautiful, and they, um, your life is better because of your loved one with a disability. And yes, there is value, there is not a burden, you know what I mean? You just want to clarify that.

One interpretation of this statement is as an example of what disability activist Stella Young dubbed "inspiration porn," a pervasive and objectifying perspective that disability exists to teach nondisabled people lessons about gratitude, tenacity, and humanity.[8] Disabled children's value, in this construction, comes from their ability to enrich the lives of others, not from their intrinsic being. Anton shared a similar perspective when discussing the potential of PGT to eliminate certain kinds of people from the world:

> Well, you might say that's a good thing, but what do you learn from someone with [cystic fibrosis]? You can learn a lot of things from them. You can learn a lot about human nature, and um, overcoming great obstacles and difficult things. I mean, they teach us a lot about who we are as—people who go through different struggles teach us a lot. So, I'm afraid we'll become boring.

Again, nondisabled rather than disabled experiences and desires are centered, and the value of disability emerges from what a disabled person can teach nondisabled people.

Not all of the informants' perspectives on disability as valuable were inflected with inspiration porn, however. Patsy, Melanie, and

Abby all had personal and professional relationships with disabled people that informed their opinions. Patsy noted that she resented the implication that disability or ill health immediately invalidates someone's worth:

> I guess I don't like the connotation that if you're not healthy, you're not able to, you know, make a contribution to society or you know have a meaningful full life. I guess that's kind of the big picture.

Authority and Optionality in Pursuit of Responsible Parenthood

Many of the prospective parents and professionals considered PGT an essential act in the performance of responsible pregnancy management—and therefore, responsible parenthood. In this section, I consider the ways in which responsibility manifests through the perceived obligation to act and the subsequent blame applied to prospective parents. Melanie's experience exemplifies this feeling of obligation. She told me that when she was presented with information about PGT very early in her first pregnancy at an obstetrician appointment, she felt that she was being forced into a position of responsibility that she had anticipated having more time to prepare for:

> So, when they do all of this, are giving you so much risk stuff that it's like, as I'm about to be a new mom and you already make very tough decisions about your child when the child is just a fetus at that point. Like, I already had the maternal feelings, but I didn't have the feelings of like this as a child and this is what this means to make decisions. You think you're going to have to make those decisions when the baby is born. I had to start making decisions when the baby was still in the womb.

"Why Would You Say No to Your Doctor?": The Obligation to Act

For both the prospective parents and the clinicians, performing parenthood responsibly often meant that because testing is available, parents are obligated to pursue it. Not obtaining information, regardless of how it might or might not affect decision-making, was viewed as reckless. "I had to prove that I'm going to do everything I can if it's going to be something wrong or whatever," Abby told me. She felt compelled to demonstrate her fitness for motherhood and implicitly linked preparedness with the knowledge accumulation that comes from genetic screening. Gene, too, felt an obligation to test, noting simply, "Some stuff you want to take off the table. In terms of the ultimate goal of providing the start of a long, healthy, and happy life." Interestingly, when pressed about what was screened for, he replied that he "didn't know much of the ins and outs . . . you could test for other, more common issues. Down syndrome and the like." His relative lack of knowledge about what it was that screening could "take off the table" reveals an implicit trust that clinical and commercial interests matched his own, and that there is no disagreement about what kinds of conditions or genetic anomalies interfere with a good quality of life. In all cases, the prospective parents felt that if they declined testing, they would be jeopardizing the health of their future children.

An additional dimension of the perceived obligation to pursue testing came from the authority or credibility of the medical professional recommending the procedure. While some prospective parents outright rejected the notion of feeling pressured to perform PGT—as Rosalie stated, "I didn't feel like it was a requirement"—the majority of both prospective parents and professionals alluded to the distinct power dynamic that emerges when a medical professional recommends a procedure. Genetic counselor Marcie most bluntly acknowledged this fact when discussing noninvasive prenatal testing specifically:

> It's coercive. "Have this blood test done and it will tell you if your baby's okay." Absolutely! They're not given a choice. No, that's not true, they do say, "You can." But without the explanation, it's your doctor saying, it's the authority saying. Why would you say no to your doctor?

Clinicians Julia, Carmen, Miriam, and Anton all felt their role as genetic counselors included reaffirming the optionality of screening and testing, as they all had encountered prospective parents who interpreted their physicians' recommendations as mandatory.

As Carmen shared, prospective parents often enter into conversation with a genetic counselor suspiciously:

> I do think that there's a good number of people that just assume that if you talk to a genetic counselor, we're going to tell you to terminate your baby. You know, it's because there's something wrong and we're going to tell you to terminate.

She later described how she approaches these difficult interactions, noting that emphasizing the prospective parent's autonomy often serves to establish a working relationship. "I've had other patients that seem like they've warmed up to me," she said, "as soon as I told them that these testing options were, in fact, optional." Importantly, informants who noted this phenomenon often suggested it was rooted in poor clinical communication rather than in misunderstanding on the part of the prospective parent. In fact, in many instances, genetic counselors articulated a somewhat combative relationship with other clinicians, aligning themselves both implicitly and explicitly with the desires and well-being of the prospective parent. The prospective parents interviewed, however, did not report this kind of relationship.

All the reviewed documentation in some way touched on the responsibility of prospective parents, whether it was their responsibility to prepare adequately for pregnancy and child-rearing, their responsibility for communicating with their family members, or their responsibility to request a specific brand of PGT from their clinicians. Primarily, these documents presented PGT as a necessary step for responsible parenthood. Documentation was also embedded with rhetoric suggesting that prospective parents have an obligation to act in the pursuit of knowledge. Screening was almost universally presented in terms of providing knowledge to prepare for a disabled child, with results being described as "actionable" or "of clinical significance" and next steps often including finding specialists and establishing a care plan. One commercial website read, for example, "Having information about these chromosomal changes before birth can help ensure your baby receives the proper and necessary support." Only one-third of the sources reviewed mentioned termination as an option following testing, and even then, it was often referenced obliquely as an "irreversible" pregnancy management decision. The emphasis on PGT as essential for preparing for the birth of a nonnormative child encodes the responsibility of the parents: Without testing, they are not providing appropriate care and support. Here, choice (including the choice to terminate) is minimized in favor of a discourse of personal responsibility toward a future child. It should be noted that the majority of documents were directed specifically at women, reinforcing a gendered dimension of responsible parenthood echoed in some interviews.

Further, all written sources used the term "baby" or "unborn baby," as opposed to "fetus," when discussing PGT, suggesting the existence of a parental relationship prior to birth, and thus reaffirming parental responsibility. Use of the term "baby" and the absence of rhetorics of choice, one clinician pointed out to me upon reading an initial draft of this chapter, may not be intended to promote ideas of parental responsibility at all; rather, the language might be demanded by external factors, such as the need to write accessibly for a general audience and restrictions on abortion in parts of the United States. The impact of these discourses, however, is not dependent on their intentionality. This emotive language in official documents, especially those used by prospective parents for decision-making, requires a deeper analysis.

Elsewhere, however, the optionality of testing was emphasized, creating a curious juxtaposition with the framing described above. One source's FAQs stated, "All testing is optional. The decision to accept or decline screening is a personal choice and should be one you discuss with your healthcare provider." The majority of the documentation, particularly that coming from commercial testing companies, implied that prospective parents have a significant number of choices as to the types and brands of testing they receive, often encouraging them to request one specific company's test over another's. However, the majority of prospective parents I spoke with did not even know which company's tests were being used until after they received their results. Rather, the tests were chosen by the clinics they visited, with little attention paid, in the clinical interaction, to the details of the private companies involved. Further, guidance documents often stated that PGT is part of routine care, such as one professional society informational page that read, "Both screening and diagnostic testing are offered to all pregnant women." The routinization of procedures such as PGT inherently affects their perceived optionality.[9]

"I've Been Told That I Need to Be More Grateful": Disrupted Joy

In addition to a sense of obligation to pursue screening in order to perform parenthood responsibly, the majority of prospective parents also noted that the imposition of screening and testing, a topic often broached during the first obstetrician appointment, created additional anxiety, disrupted their ability to celebrate, or alienated them from the pregnancy. This created distinct "before" and "after" periods, marking when they could accept the reality of the future child. Rosalie's experience strongly resembled what Barbara Katz Rothman described as a "tentative pregnancy" more than thirty years ago.[10] Rosalie told me:

> The day that I got the genetic test results it sort of allowed me to own it. And really feel like a pregnant woman who is having a baby. Like a future mother. I hadn't really—I think I sort of didn't allow myself to integrate that identity because I was so afraid that something bad was going to happen that I was going to have to terminate or, you know, miscarry or something awful or some awful result. So, for me, just emotionally, that was sort of like a milestone.

At the time of the interviews, none of the genetic counselors discussed the disruption caused by PGT, but one clinician commented on an initial draft of this chapter to confirm that this theme also resonated with her experience:

> I very frequently share my experience (when educating other providers, usually) that giving a patient "bad news" (at any point on the spectrum from there may be a problem/background risk to we know there is a problem/diagnosis) creates a tremendous disruption in the pregnancy experience. One that can really NEVER be resolved. That dose of reality (again, wherever it falls on the spectrum) against the expectation is shocking. I did this countless times to my patients. The best counselor in the world can't avoid the disruption, but there are certainly ways to do it better.

As described earlier in this chapter, Melanie, who had previous reproductive issues that made her unsure she could even conceive, felt she was immediately thrust into the position of making life-altering decisions around her fetus's health: "So we didn't really get to celebrate because all of us sudden all these questions got brought to us."

The liminality of pregnancy—the simultaneous presence and absence of the fetus—also affected how the prospective parents and clinicians understood their relationship to disability. Abby, for example, stated, "When you're pregnant, you don't know your baby as a person yet. So, when you get a diagnosis, it's easier, I think, to just think of them as just the diagnosis, because they're not people." Sabrina, a clinical scientist and researcher, also noted prospective parents' tendency or ability to abstract their pregnancy in a way they could not with a child. She shared a study suggesting that, rather than making it easier to terminate, as Abby thought, this kind of abstraction could eventually empower prospective parents to pursue in utero therapeutic options.[11] Describing the study's findings, she said:

> [Prospective parents] stated that it was important that their unborn child didn't yet have a personality. Once a child was born, that child (he or she) existed as they were, and they loved them for who they were. But when the child was still in utero, they felt that treatment was okay. They wanted to do whatever they could to help the child because they really didn't know what the child would be like. I think that it was very interesting that that distinction was made.

Rosalie, Melanie, and Abby all shared that they felt an obligation to shield others in their lives from the anxiety and stress they experienced during their pregnancies, and this led to feelings of isolation. Only Rosalie, however, connected her anxiety directly to genetic testing: "I was afraid to tell anyone because if God forbid something awful were to come of it, I didn't want to have to explain to so many people that something terrible happened when they were so excited." Her isolation was exacerbated by feelings of guilt and responsibility, which she recognized as related to her unique, gendered position as the carrier of the pregnancy:

> So, I was lonely. And it sucked and because my partner wasn't really worried about that kind of stuff, I kind of felt like I was on

> my own in it. . . . Yeah, you know, I think people really want to be excited. . . . It just felt like, you know, I don't want him to be super stoked that I'm having a baby and then me just rain on the whole parade and say that I'm so afraid of all these things.

Part of this impulse to shield others from anxiety and stress seemed to emerge, at least for Melanie and Abby, from perceived judgment from others who suggested they were not sufficiently grateful for their pregnancies. "I've been told that I need to be more grateful," Melanie recalled. When she would express to others how difficult her pregnancy was, she was told that "it's not fair for me to be so upset when there's other people who can't have kids." The implication that pregnant people may not feel welcome to express their concerns or anxieties suggests a form of epistemic invalidation that delegitimates the experiences of pregnant people who have not fulfilled the impossible standard of an ideal pregnancy. When I asked Abby what a "healthy pregnancy" meant to her, she recounted the difficulty of comparing her own pregnancy, which involved fertility treatments prior to conception, with her vision of a healthy pregnancy, or "when you just get pregnant the way you're supposed to and then things develop how they're supposed to, and you never have complications. . . . It's the dream world of having a baby."

In describing this nearly unattainable ideal, Abby positioned not only her pregnancy but nearly every other pregnancy as pathologized. More broadly, medical intervention of almost any kind is often seen as disrupting the "naturalness" of pregnancy, with medicalization equated to unhealthiness. Rosalie and Melanie also pathologized their pregnancies (Rosalie's as geriatric, Melanie's as complicated by her own health issues). This pathologization reinforced their feelings of guilt and shame as they fell short of an unattainable ideal.

Additional common experiences among prospective parents linked to their perceptions of responsible parenthood were feelings of blame, guilt, and judgment, directed either at themselves or at other prospective parents. Abby expressed judgment toward other prospective parents who used access to PGT results in ways that were vastly different from what she herself would have done. She recalled reading a post in an online pregnancy forum by another prospective parent who decided to terminate a pregnancy that had a positive diagnosis for a genetic disorder. "I guess it's hard when you see it," she told me:

> Because I'm like, "I wanted that baby." It's not even my baby . . . I think it's just hard for me, especially because of what I went through. I want these babies so badly, no matter what, that . . . I don't want to say I feel judgmental, but I kind of do. I'm just angered by it, I guess, because I'm like, why would you be proud of [termination]?

Genetic counselor Julia also struggled with recognizing and withholding judgment of others, particularly when her personal beliefs and her professional obligation to be a "nondirective counselor" were at odds:

> You have to buy into [nondirectiveness]. You really do. But you really have to appreciate that you have to let people do what they're comfortable doing. And it really doesn't have anything to do with "what you would do, if . . ." And over the years, people have made decisions that I would never do if it was me. Never, ever. But it's not me.

Genetic counselor Anton also emphasized the complexity of needing to remove his own beliefs about disability from his work:

> And so, it's not as easy as just, I think that everybody has, you know, intrinsic value and they should be valued, and you should go on and you should deliver every baby with a problem. Um, whether you think that or not, it's much more complicated, because not everybody is going to be able to carry that baby to term, and so there's a lot more that goes into it than just, how you feel about whether a person does termination or not.

Taken together, these examples of judgment of others reveal that each informant was operating with an implicit framework about the "correct" use of the knowledge acquired from PGT, and that different frameworks are often at odds.

While the documents examined often advocated for understanding and weighing the risks of prenatal genetic testing, they rarely mentioned the affective experiences articulated here. Almost universally, commercial companies promoted noninvasive testing, emphasizing the physical risk of miscarriage with other testing methods (such as amniocentesis) and describing NIPS as “simple” and safe, with no physical risk to “mother and child.” Only two of the sources reviewed, from a health system and a professional society, suggested that there are nonphysical risks associated with genetic testing that may need to be considered. As the health system’s informational page noted, “Genetic testing can have emotional, social and financial risks as well.” This source also briefly addressed discrimination and stigma associated with genetic conditions, as well as legal recourse under the Genetic Information Nondiscrimination Act (GINA). While other documentation discussed some of the elements of responsible parenthood brought up by informants, many of the personal and emotional difficulties experienced by prospective parents—including overwhelming clinical experiences, testing’s disruption of their joy in pregnancy, and feelings of guilt and judgment—were predictably absent from these documents.

In Pursuit of Responsible Parenthood: Knowing and Acting with Prenatal Genetic Testing

In this chapter, I untangle the messy relationships among prenatal genetic testing, knowledge accumulation, and responsible pregnancy management under neoliberal conditions. Prospective parents are subject to impossible expectations: They must act as fully autonomous agential responsible citizens while simultaneously deferring to clinical authority; they are “fully informed” but also reliant on the partial framing of disability presented in prenatal care settings. Prospective parents are faced with the increasing routinization of prenatal testing in obstetrics care, paired with an illusion of certainty in testing results. These factors create conditions under which the performance of informed consent cannot be truly informed. In this section, I first grapple with how gender and class mediated the experiences of my informants. Next, I argue that the pressures of neoliberal responsible citizenship and the moral imperative to adopt technology disallow nonparticipation in PGT. I then show that seeking either too much or too little knowledge about future children through genetic testing is perceived as a moral transgression, before turning to the conspicuous absence of embodied knowledge in PGT development and use.

Gender, Class, and Performing Responsibility

By most accounts, nearly every pregnant person in the United States seeking obstetric care is now offered prenatal genetic screening. The interviews presented in this chapter cannot and do not seek to be representative of that enormous and diverse population. While diverse in terms of geographic location, those featured here shared some key similarities: all were white, middle- to upper-middle-class, with higher education and stable employment. Nearly all identified as women. The clinicians and genetic professionals interviewed also largely mirrored these characteristics. I believe, as I describe in this section, that these characteristics inflect the informants' encounters with PGT in meaningful ways, and that these prospective parents and professionals are, in fact, representative of a population commonly targeted by the PGT apparatus. As Marsha Saxton writes, in rejection of the argument that controversies around selective abortion harm nonprivileged women by eliminating choice for already choice-constrained populations:

> It is the middle and upper class who most often can purchase these "reproductive choices." It's not poor women, or families with problematic genetic traits, who are creating the market for tests. Women with aspirations for the "perfect baby" are establishing new "standards of care." Responding to the lure of consumerism, they are helping create a lucrative market that exploits the culture's fear of disability and makes huge profits for the biotech industry.[12]

There is a rich history of feminist scholarship attending to the specific pressures of accountability placed on cisgender women of childbearing age.[13] I too note gendered dimensions throughout informants' descriptions of their experiences, from common references to "mothers" (as opposed to "parents") to several instances in which embodied and experiential knowledge was linked explicitly to femaleness. Only two informants—one prospective parent and one genetic counselor—identified as male. Perspectives in this case were also dominated by a heterosexism that assumed a pregnant person to be in a male–female relationship, even as pregnant informants themselves were uncoupled or identified as queer. Similarly, there were assumptions akin to a biological essentialism that viewed good or responsible motherhood (not parenthood) as a biologically innate characteristic. Further, class and educational dimensions appeared explicitly throughout the case. Genetic counseling professionals often alluded to a certain type of prospective parent suggestive of a wealthy, educated person who, in Marcie's words, lives in an urban area and "want[s] a perfect baby."[14] Suggestions of regionality as factoring into health literacy and ultimately into trust of genetic screening and testing also point to how class, race, and ethnicity inflect decisions around prenatal testing. As Miriam told me:

> I think on the East Coast and on the West Coast, it might—kind of the genome and those more—screening for things that maybe people aren't at risk for is a little bit bigger, but I think generally in the Midwest, we have less uptake on even things like carrier screening for cystic fibrosis. We just have less uptake, it feels like. So, I anticipate that it's already different based on location, part of those conversations with geneticists.

Rosalie explicitly addressed how her reproductive anxieties emerged directly from her class; she currently placed herself in the "middle class," juxtaposing it with what she described as a working-class upbringing. In her current class, not only was she part of a generation of women giving birth in their mid-thirties, but also "this demographic, you know, there's so much pressure on parents to be perfect and to be great and everything that their kid does reflects on them as a person. . . . There definitely is a lot of ownership in parenting in this class that I feel like in the lower class that I came from, it's just a different thing. You don't own it the same way."[15] This differential understanding of the expectations of motherhood bled into perceptions of pregnancy, including responsibility for congenital disability.

On a more fundamental level, Alison Kafer asserts that the figure of the Child—the metaphoric symbol of future humanity—is used to maintain expectations of nondisabledness and heteronormativity in a variety of social and cultural settings. Therefore, certain conditions detected by prenatal testing are understood as threats to the figure of the Child and to the future of humans more broadly. Kafer suggests that the proliferation of prenatal testing technologies is tightly coupled with "profound anxieties about reproducing the family as a normative unit."[16] "Normative," in this context, refers not only to nondisabledness but also to heterosexuality, socioeconomic security, and whiteness.[17] There is intense social pressure for prospective parents—primarily prospective mothers—to use these technologies appropriately, and failure to reproduce the idealized Child results in stigmatization. Therefore, it is impossible to discuss the meaning of the ableism embedded in prenatal genetic testing without also attending to the gendered, racialized, and heterosexist dimensions that animate genetic screening and testing in theory and practice.

Naturalizing and Obscuring the Moral Imperative

In the informants' accounts of their personal experiences, as well as in the analyzed guidance documents, the role of genetic testing in prenatal and preimplantation care was taken for granted. Melanie's recollection of being encouraged to attend genetic counseling while receiving a pelvic exam during her first obstetrics appointment exemplifies the ways in which genetic testing—and the assumption of the necessity of knowledge accumulation that accompanies it—has become naturalized into health care services. Therefore, the implications of genetic testing have become obscured. Despite the ostensible optionality of screening and testing, the routinization of these strategies, alongside the perceived power imbalance between expert clinicians and prospective parents, may constitute a form of coercion.[18] As Marcie commented, "Why would you say no to your doctor?" The settled nature of this case, in which PGT is integrated as a routine element of obstetric care, raises further questions about informed autonomous decision-making. Prospective parents are expected to make decisions based on partial, highly medicalized information, with little institutional support and increasing pressure to pursue technological intervention.[19] We can see this particularly in the failure to articulate all possibilities for (non)intervention. As Annette Patterson and Martha Satz write, "Increasingly, obstetricians do not 'offer' pregnant women prenatal testing. . . . Women often undergo such testing without becoming fully aware that they may refuse to do so."[20] Further, the legal and political grounding for informed consent is the concept of the "reasonable actor" capable of neutral, unemotional, and detached decision-making.[21] However, such an actor does not exist. What information is relevant for decision-making, what factors influence how and when a person pursues intervention, what framework a person uses to decide—these elements are highly individualized and contextual, and their consideration may be "reasonable only to [the person] himself or herself."[22] The knowledge tensions that undoubtedly affect how "informed" consent can truly be are illustrated by Abby's frustration with her clinician's unwillingness to discuss next steps before the completion of genetic testing, by Julia's acknowledgment that prospective parents want to know if a future child will be able to work or live on their own, and by the different frameworks through which clinicians discuss disability.

At the same time, the pressures to perform responsible citizenship animate logics in the prenatal clinic. This discourse is particularly forceful when applied to biotechnological intervention on nonnormative bodyminds. As Sarah Franklin writes in reference to fertility technologies, "There is no sense of choice or options within this depiction of scientific progress: it is as eventually inevitable as it is morally imperative to proceed forward."[23] Rather than being encouraged to manage disease and disability as they desire, individuals are expected to approximate a nondisabled ideal. Michael Bérubé provides a similar commentary on the pressures of good citizenship faced by parents of children (or prospective children) with disabilities, arguing that families "must be protected from state coercion yet supported by the state's apparatus of social welfare."[24] Diane Paul writes extensively about the tensions between individual and public health models of care, noting that they are inherently in conflict. The former concerns itself with autonomy and the agency of the individual to make any choice, while the latter is concerned with the common good and the individual's responsibility toward it.[25] An extreme but poignant example of this tension coming to a head is the involuntary sterilization of people with intellectual disabilities, people with mental illness, and others who were categorized as "unfit" in the early and mid-twentieth century in the United States. These individuals often wished to bear and raise children (and some had), but the hegemonic eugenic discourse of the day argued that their autonomy needed to be restricted for the sake of cultivating a civilized public sphere.[26] In the case of present-day genetic testing, while much has been written about nondirectiveness and parental autonomy at the level of the clinic, as Paul observes in a discussion of state-funded screening and testing, "that the state expects to save money is evident in the arguments actually made to legislatures, which are typically framed in cost-benefit terms."[27]

Knowledge Transgressions

Rayna Rapp articulates the double weight placed on women of childbearing age, who are both scrutinized and surveilled while simultaneously singularly burdened with choice: They are "culturally positioned to think about their reproductive capacities, desires, and decisions as a private dimension of public life."[28] Pregnant people are forced into the role of "moral pioneer," deciding which children are eligible to enter their communities. In other words, the introduction of these new technologies creates responsibilities that pregnant people are expected to navigate in a way that satisfies both their private and their public duties. They become enmeshed in a technoscientific apparatus with profound reproductive consequences. Rapp concludes by asserting that there is a need to interrogate the social alongside the biomedical:

> Women are both constrained and empowered through technologies like amniocentesis to serve as our contemporary moral pioneers. At once held accountable at the individual level for a cascade of broadly social factors which shape the health outcome of each pregnancy, and individually empowered to decide whether and when there are limits on voluntary parenthood, women offered an amniocentesis are also philosophers and gatekeepers of the limits of who may join our current communities.[29]

Notable here also is what knowledge is absent from these interactions. A strange disembodiment infuses understandings of disability in PGT development and use. The visualization of trisomy in a karyotype or the material experience of drawing blood to test genetic material in NIPS seems in some way to solidify disability as materially real. The presence or absence of genetic difference makes disability a tangible reality: detectable and therefore preventable. At the same time, because of the inherent presence/absence of the fetus, the future disabled child is itself abstracted. As demonstrated through informants' descriptions of their experiences, both prospective parents and medical professionals have next to no exposure to embodied experiences of disability. Embodied knowledge is not considered part of the essential knowledge acquired through PGT.

Through the process of screening for disability, a fetus of uncertain status becomes a future child. The slippage between "fetus" and "baby" in guidance documents and clinical conversations has consequences. Saxton notes how this rhetorical sleight of hand moves in the opposite direction when PGT yields a result suggesting disability: "Fetuses that are wanted are called 'babies.' Prenatal screening results can turn a 'wanted baby' into an 'unwanted fetus.'" She also calls attention to reticence among medical professionals to label a fetus itself as "disabled." Instead, the language of positive probabilities, chromosomal differences, and specific diagnoses tends to proliferate. To label a fetus disabled, she argues, "we personify the fetus via a term of pride in the disability community. The fetus is named as a member of our community." Saxton draws attention to an inherent, if unspoken, conflict within communities fighting for reproductive justice. "It is important," she writes, "to make the distinction between a pregnant woman who chooses to terminate the pregnancy because she doesn't want to be pregnant as opposed to a pregnant woman who wanted to be pregnant but rejects a particular fetus, a particular potential child."[30] Yet this distinction is completely invisible in both informant interviews and guidance documents. The rhetoric of choice looms large across this case, and yet, as Alexandra Minna Stern concludes, women of childbearing age are caught in a medical and moral dilemma in which they are "pulled betwixt and between the seeming autonomy of choice, diminishing reproductive control, and the burden of receiving consequential medical and genetic knowledge."[31] The intractable tensions between the rhetorics of individual autonomy and the public good trap prospective parents under the weight of impossible expectations.

The tacit assumption that genetic knowledge about some conditions, like Down syndrome, is necessary for pregnancy management while other knowledge may lead to unnecessary anxiety suggests that some conditions are inherently less desirable. It is unclear in the interviews what makes Down syndrome significantly less desirable than any one of the single-gene anomalies detected through a full panel, although its prominence in prenatal testing may be due in part simply to its relative ease of detection. Unlike trisomy 13 and trisomy 18, which are also screened for in most standard screenings, Down syndrome does not typically cause death in early childhood. It is possible, however, that familiarity with Down syndrome leads both prospective parents and professionals to believe that detection and intervention are necessary. However, the taken-for-grantedness of PGT—and of the inherent undesirability of conditions commonly screened for—prevents these types of questions from surfacing in most clinical interactions.

Further, some informants, like Rosalie, expressed that the knowledge acquired during PGT made their pregnancies—and their future children—more real. But what makes the karyotype of an additional copy of a chromosome more real than the testimony of adults with Down syndrome about their quality of life? Elizabeth Barnes argues that the deeply rooted belief among nondisabled populations that disability is inherently "bad-difference," as opposed to "mere-difference," means that when disabled people express that they are satisfied, they are immediately cast as unreliable witnesses in their own lives.[32] Bioethicist Jackie Leach Scully suspects this disbelief stems from an assumption that disabled people's positive perceptions of their lives "are inherently untrustworthy and possibly self-serving in a way that those of nondisabled people are not."[33] The epistemic invalidation of embodied and experiential knowledge is so total here that in some ways, disabled people have been erased entirely from PGT.

Integrating embodied disabled knowledge into PGT could change not just how decision-making around PGT occurs but also the nature and scope of what is considered reasonable and responsible to genetically test for in the first place. We have the technological capability to test the entire genome. Embodied disabled knowledge could inform the decisions we make about what we find meaningful to develop testing for, and what we integrate into standard practice. For example, currently the National Society of Genetic Counselors recommends against using predictive genetic testing on minors for adult-onset conditions "until the individual has the capacity to weigh the associated risks, benefits, and limitations of this information, taking his/her circumstances, preferences, and beliefs into account to preserve his/her autonomy and right to an open future."[34] As can be seen here, best practices in genetic counseling already emphasize choice, autonomy, and opportunity, and yet the "right to an open future" is one conspicuously absent for potential children with congenital disabilities. How does "childhood management" of disability, to use the terminology of the National Society of Genetic Counselors, so dramatically shift the scope of parental authority? At its root, the answer lies in the perceived desirability of disabled lives. Would acknowledging—and believing—what congenitally disabled people say about their lives change the scope of what prenatal genetic testing is perceived as meaningful or necessary?

Prospective parents are subject to contradictory pressures in the construction of responsible parenthood through the knowledge acquired in prenatal genetic testing. Each choice in pregnancy management is scrutinized and moralized. Prospective parents are perceived as transgressing if they fail to know through a refusal of genetic information, as well as if they fail to defer to clinical authority regarding the parameters of what constitutes the "right knowledge" for making responsible and informed decisions. As evidenced by the interviews quoted above, prospective parents feel judged for an "immoral refusal to exercise autonomy," to borrow Melinda Hall's phrasing, when they resist engaging with genetic technologies.[35] As Abby alluded to when wrestling with the decision herself, refusal to engage with medical technologies is interpreted as a failure to act in the future child's best interests. Choosing to reject the necessity of genetic knowledge is perceived as negligence. At the same time, the existence of genetic knowledge as a result of testing requires action on the part of the prospective parent, who must make choices that otherwise would not be demanded. As Melanie recalled, "You think you're going to have to make those decisions when the baby is born. I had to start making decisions when the baby was still in the womb." At the same time prospective parents are expected to be responsible and informed actors, they are also expected to defer to the authority of the clinician. While medical professionals rely on biomedical or physiological definitions, obfuscating the social, embodied, and experiential dimensions of disability, prospective parents are expected to make "fully informed" autonomous decisions in contexts where they express lacking crucial information. Medical professionals have established their authority to determine what nonprofessionals should know (and what is "too much" knowledge), nearly always classifying social and embodied knowledge as superfluous. This arrangement creates conditions under which undesirable pregnancy outcomes are naturalized. In other words, the conditions detected through recommended genetic screens and tests are assumed to be undesirable, regardless of the prospective parents' actual understanding of the conditions or the technologies. Additionally, the complicated relationship between medical authority and perceptions of personal, parental, and social responsibility comes to bear on the decision to pursue testing. Ultimately, these findings indicate several sites of tension in the PGT apparatus, from disjunctions in how, when, and to whom information is communicated to the conflict between the perceived obligatory nature of screening and explicit statements of optionality and agency. The following chapter, which considers how disablement and the pressures of neoliberal ableism complicate the experience of choosing and using deep brain stimulation, continues to think through agency and accountability while exploring how transgressions of expertise and the body itself create credibility contests in the clinic and beyond.

« 3 »

Losing and Taking Control with Deep Brain Stimulation

In the summer of 2019, I spoke to Carl, a middle-aged man living in the Midwest. A few years earlier, Carl had a small device implanted in his brain to manage the symptoms of dystonia, a kind of involuntary muscle contraction. While this process, called deep brain stimulation, did relieve pain and dystonia symptoms, shortly after Carl received the implant he began experiencing auditory hallucinations. He told me he often heard the voices of his care team at the hospital where he had his implant surgery. To him, that was no coincidence. He believed his hallucinations stemmed from his use of his patient remote to adjust the DBS's settings. Despite the fact that the patient remote is designed to provide some latitude for users to adjust stimulator settings within preset parameters, Carl felt that in doing so he had taken action outside his role as a passive recipient of technology. In other words, he had transgressed the boundary between patient and clinician. He asserted that he should not be "making my own adjustments, because I'm not a neurologist."

Despite increasing evidence that deep brain stimulation can cause both acute and persistent mental health symptoms, Carl's neurologist denied that the psychiatric symptoms he was having were caused by his implant. Carl was eventually involuntarily institutionalized. When speaking about that time, he consistently expressed that he was deeply affected by both the invalidation of his experiences and the lack of transparency in communication with his neurology team. He told me:

> And what really made me mad . . . I was having side effects and . . . I should be seeing my neurologist. And not be, you know,

> sentenced to an area as a guinea pig where they just, in my opinion, dope you up on pills to see if it would help your issues, like mental issues that you're having, when I knew inside that this was a side effect from the deep brain stimulation. . . . Well, when I did bring it to my neurologist and told her that, she said, quote-unquote, "That's impossible."

He wished that he had been better informed of the potential risks of his implant. The invalidation of his psychiatric symptoms made him feel isolated:

> Because that's all I wanted to hear from them was why wasn't anything said that "Hey by the way . . . you know what, Carl? After you had the surgery you might have some side effects, but that's just the trade-off and there's nothing we can do about it." I probably would have been totally cool about it. You know, I would've been much more ready for it. So, I didn't feel like I was alienated and losing my mind.

Through tears, he shared his distress about visiting his neurologist, because "she doesn't believe me. It's very upsetting. She thinks I'm crazy."

Rooting my analysis in interviews with DBS users and their partners (many of whom were also acting as caregivers) and user-directed documentation from hospital systems and clinics, I argue in this chapter that the design, use, and discourse around deep brain stimulation configures disability as a purely physiological phenomenon in need of biomedical intervention, albeit one resulting in social stigma.[1] Once disability is firmly located within the individual, perceptions of personal responsibility to manage it—particularly the elements of disability that impede economic or social productivity—emerge as central to decision-making. Additionally, people with DBS often face epistemic invalidation or dismissal when their embodied experiences challenge clinical authority in some way, often through physical, neurological, or psychiatric symptoms related to either the precipitating condition or the implant. Below, following a brief overview of expectations and outcomes related to DBS, I highlight three key characteristics that shape the experience of choosing and using deep brain stimulation. First, variable processes of meaning making produce conflicting definitions of disability and different acceptable interventions. Second, pressures for prospective users to practice self-management and control lead to the moralization of the decision to pursue DBS. Finally, tactics of credibility building in clinical settings create contexts in which embodied knowledge is invalidated, ignored, or dismissed when it comes into conflict with clinical authority. I conclude the chapter by contextualizing these experiences, arguing that while deep brain stimulation operates under a rhetoric of empowerment and control—one that is rooted in gendered expectations—that control is ultimately restricted both by epistemic invalidation and by systemic pressures of neoliberal ableism and compulsory able-bodiedness.

Intervening on the Brain

Deep brain stimulation has a wide range of applications, but in all cases it serves as a means of symptom management rather than as a cure for an underlying condition. While Carl received DBS for dystonia, most available research has been conducted with people with Parkinson's disease. A recent meta-analysis of eight studies conducted in the United Kingdom with a total of nearly 1,200 participants found that DBS for advanced Parkinson's disease resulted in improved outcomes in terms of "mental status, behavior, mood (UPDRS-I), ADLs [activities of daily living] (UPDRS-II), motor function (UPDRS-III), and complications from therapy (UPDRS-IV) in PD users" as compared to the best available medical therapy.[2] Frederick Hitti and colleagues found during a retrospective analysis of 320 American users that while DBS does not halt the progression of Parkinson's, for many it provides symptomatic relief (and user satisfaction) for at least ten years.[3] Additional research in the United States suggests DBS may be linked to longer survival rates for people with Parkinson's, in comparison to the rates for those who manage their condition with medication.[4]

However, while most studies have found that the majority of DBS users experience positive outcomes in terms of clinical symptoms and quality of life, the minority who do not is substantial. A 2016 qualitative systematic review found that studies in Denmark, France, and Sweden reported up to 43 percent of users showed no improvement in quality of life after DBS, with some reporting a decline.[5] Less than half of the recipients of DBS and their spouses perceived DBS as having resulted in a positive outcome. Importantly, these perceptions do not necessarily hinge on symptom mitigation. Franziska Maier and colleagues, studying recipients of subthalamic deep brain stimulation for Parkinson's disease in Germany in 2016, found that nearly 60 percent of participants held either negative or mixed views about their outcomes, regardless of whether the implant improved their motor symptoms.[6] These responses were linked to perceived quality of life (including levels of medication needed postimplant), mental state, and social interactions. Malco Rossi and colleagues attribute these disappointments to "unrealistic expectations" on the part of recipients of DBS, especially as these related to how DBS would affect "professional life, activities of daily living, marital relations, and social adjustments."[7] Regardless of the root cause, these statistics reveal a mismatch between what the discourse around DBS promises and what DBS actually delivers.

The scope and severity of side effects from DBS can be hard to predict from user to user, in part because side effects can be difficult to untangle from symptoms of the targeted condition. Markus Christen and colleagues note that cataloging the side effects of DBS is particularly complicated, in part because alternative therapeutic approaches, such as medication, may have similar side effects, and in part because "the evaluation of some side effects differs significantly between patients, their relatives, and physicians."[8] Nonetheless, the American Association of Neurological Surgeons (AANS) details a wide array of side effects related to DBS, ranging from those caused by the surgical implantation to those emerging from the placement of the leads in the brain tissue or exposure to electrical stimulation. Regarding the former, the AANS reports there is a 2–3 percent chance of brain hemorrhage, potentially leading to paralysis, stroke, or speech impairment; a 15 percent chance of a temporary minor implantation problem such as infection, which may result in the removal of the leads; and a very small risk of cerebrospinal fluid leakage, resulting in meningitis or headaches.[9] According to Donatus Cyron, other side effects related to the surgery itself include temporary swelling at the implantation site, tingling in the face or limbs, and allergic reaction to the implant.[10] Stimulation- or lead-related effects may include confusion, hallucinations, risk-seeking behavior, and aggression. Additional side effects include speech and vision problems, shocking sensation, loss of balance, difficulty with concentration, and dizziness.[11] Sharp increases in apathy and anxiety have been linked to certain implantation sites, as have cognitive changes.[12] According to the AANS, most of these side effects are both mild and reversible. The risk of a "serious adverse event" with DBS, however, is more than double the risk of such an event associated with the best medical therapy.[13]

Frederic Gilbert and colleagues, in reporting on a small set of semistructured interviews they conducted with seventeen recipients of DBS for Parkinson's, note that while neuropsychiatric changes caused by implants are increasingly detected and reversible, far less attention has been paid to phenomenological effects—or how users view and understand themselves. In their study, nearly all of the informants experienced shifts in how they perceived themselves following their implantation. For some, this included a deterioration in the sense of self, often linked to a perceived loss of control; others expressed feelings of restoration linked to their perception of their capacities.[14] Some recipients felt a sense of empowerment when they viewed DBS as an integrated part of themselves rather than as an invasive technology taking control. While I do not address this phenomenological framework explicitly, I too am concerned with how users perceive themselves and their relationship to technology and medicine in the process of receiving deep brain stimulation. Moreover, I seek to understand the relationship between medical intervention and neoliberal body management, as well as the consequences of embodied knowledge that challenges or resists medical authority. The next section presents the operationalization of disability in the context of DBS.

Making Meaning of Disability and DBS

When I first met Fred and his wife, Nora, he had been living with Parkinson's for nearly twenty years. He was diagnosed in 2004 and received DBS a decade later, but he said that he had symptoms of Parkinson's for a long time prior to his diagnosis. He spoke bluntly about his relationship to the disease and to the changes his body experienced because of it. "I still see my body quite often as the enemy," he told me, "because Parkinson's is still there. And what's worse, my body's never going to improve, year after year, it's only going to get worse." Fred's adversarial relationship with his body exemplified a common perception among informants, in which they considered themselves distinct from, and in conflict with, their disabled bodies. To Fred, DBS was another weapon in his arsenal to fight disability.

For many informants, their disability signaled a loss of control and DBS represented a method to regain it. They spoke of shifting relationships with their bodies, which in turn influenced the risks they were willing to take with them. Tensions between how clinicians viewed potential DBS users and how they viewed themselves manifested in mismatched expectations, poor or combative clinical communication, and perceived underpreparedness of the users for the physical and emotional experience of both their diagnosed condition and the DBS procedure.

"Don't Let Tremors Control Your Life": Disability as Enemy

While I spoke to people who received DBS for a number of different reasons, not limited to Parkinson's, dystonia, and chronic pain, nearly all of them had acquired disability over the course of their lives. Their descriptions of their current state often contained an understanding of disability that was directly related to a loss of function, control, or movement—in other words, a shifting away from an idealized, nondisabled body or self. George, for example, was a seventy-year-old DBS user living in the mid-Atlantic region whose Parkinson's diagnosis came from his exposure to Agent Orange during the Vietnam War. He told me that Parkinson's meant "your life changes in ways which you have no control over." The perceived inevitability of decline or impotence to prevent disease progression is exemplified in what John, a seventy-five-year-old living in Northern California who received DBS, told me, quoting a former health provider who also had Parkinson's: "It's like my old psychiatrist says, 'You know we're screwed, don't you? Grow a beard to cover the drooling.'" These users' perceptions of the disabled bodymind as out of control contributed to their desire to regain or enact control through technological intervention. Bradley, the youngest informant at thirty-four, had received DBS for chronic pain following a stroke. To him, the device restored the humanity he felt he had lost through his pain and the use of narcotics to manage it. "Now I actually feel like I felt before I had my stroke," he said. "I just feel human. So, it's just the overall comfort of it all."

This statement reveals an orientation to disability as inherently dehumanizing. Control allowed Bradley to reachieve humanity.

Examining documentation from hospital systems, neurological clinics, and medical device manufacturers, I found that nearly all these materials used language that presented disability or disease as an invasion, loss of control, or deviation from an ideal self, simultaneously figuring DBS as a means of control or return to able-bodiedness. For example, one success story on the use of DBS for dystonia published by a children's hospital described the person who received treatment as having to "fight his own limbs" prior to DBS, articulating the disabled body as separate and in conflict. Other documents framed disability as a struggle for control. "Don't let tremors control your life," read the heading on a university hospital's information page on DBS, while another hospital's interview with a neurosurgeon suggested that "patients are freed from the tremors with the flip of a switch." Rhetorically creating distance from and vilifying the nonnormative body reifies biomedical intervention as imperative for the resumption of authority over an unruly embodiment.

For Carl, the control enabled by DBS felt precarious, and he expressed a discomfort in knowing that he was beholden to a piece of technology to subdue the pain he was feeling from dystonia, sharing, "I mean, that's the scary thing too is that I'm relying on this device. It's not a cure, it helps you get through the day." Therefore, DBS represented a newfound means of control over an unruly body, but not one that originated from himself. He had to trust the technology to behave as intended; unlike Bradley, he viewed the device, not himself, as in control of his symptoms. While the control was displaced to the device, however, the responsibility for management was not. In other words, while Carl had to trust the technology to control his symptoms, he still felt personally responsible for the outcome.

The element of control enabled by DBS was acutely felt by several informants who developed infections that required removal and replacement of their devices. These informants provided a unique perspective on the sociological and psychological impacts of the perceived gain and loss of control. Fred shared the distress he experienced without his device: "I guess the simple fact is, it was terrible without it. It was a tremendous daily impact on all my life. I felt like I was circling the drain if I'm honest." He had these feelings even though, as his wife reported, the visible symptoms of Fred's Parkinson's did not reemerge as strongly as they had expected.

Lynn, who had received DBS in 2011 after living with Parkinson's for more than ten years, felt her experience of her body without DBS was magnified through the judgment she anticipated from others. She noted that "when we took out the wires, I discovered how much I tremored. And I had dyskinesia and freezing, and everything I hated about it." She elaborated, "I hated tremoring. I hated shaking. That's obvious to people." Therefore, the control she experienced was not simply control over her body but also control over her self-image. With the implant, she was able to navigate interactions without an obligation to disclose her disability through its visual dimensions, reestablishing some authority over her self-presentation.

"Why Is There Nowhere for Me to Sit Down?": The Social Dimensions of Disability

As demonstrated through Lynn's story, perceived loss of control extended not only into bodily function but also into control of self-image. Fear of appearing different, weak, or disabled was threaded throughout many of the conversations. Unaccommodating attitudes and infrastructures peppered the daily experiences of informants. Escaping these seemed in some cases to influence the decision to pursue deep brain stimulation.

For some, the difference produced through disability came to the fore when they encountered inaccessible spaces. For example, Marty, a retiree living in the Southeastern United States, recounted an incident at a local shopping center. While out shopping, he started having difficulty walking and eventually realized he would not be able to walk back to the parking lot on his own:

> And you know, when you have that—like I'm not a very self-conscious person, but like now I feel it makes me more upset when it happens because I feel like, you know, people are looking at me, I feel like, you know. So, you almost become agitated like, you know, why is there no chair? Why is there nowhere for me to sit down? You know, those kinds of things are racing through your mind.

In this situation, Marty was confronted by the construction of a material world that is not accommodating to his bodymind while simultaneously experiencing embarrassment that others were identifying him as differentially experiencing that world. Several of the documents analyzed also emphasized the social and observable dimensions of disability prior to implantation, noting that such differences could be "embarrassing," or even leave someone "emotionally traumatized."

Fred, who was highly involved as a disabled advocate in his community, shared his experience as a person with Parkinson's, speaking about attitudinal barriers arising from visual differences and also the work he does to educate others to address those barriers:

> One thing I'll say in educational talks about Parkinson's: What you see is the first thing about yourself that someone else in public notices. But what you see with Parkinson's is not what you get. What someone looks like when they have Parkinson's is not necessarily how they feel. I can't express myself the way a normal person normally does. Visual cues are off-limits with Parkinson's.

When I asked him for examples, he shared several anecdotes about people misinterpreting his body movements and assuming that he needed assistance in public settings. Both Marty and Fred emphasized the impact of others perceiving them differently because of disability or illness. They made sure to clarify, however, that this stigmatization was distinct and separate from the embodied experience of disease. Regardless of the motivation for its use—stigma or embodied need—deep brain stimulation primarily addresses the outwardly observable symptoms of conditions like Parkinson's (tremor, gait, and so on). Given the impacts of the perceptions of others and the frustrations caused by inaccessible infrastructure, such results may be viewed as significantly improving quality of life.

While visible difference was a source of tension for many informants, it was not the sum of their embodied experience. However, an overattendance to the visible aspects of disability by clinicians produced contexts in which other embodied aspects of the users' conditions were unaddressed or undervalued. As Marty shared, recounting his first visit to a support group:

> One thing that nobody ever mentioned, not once since I had this is, you know, it actually hurts sometimes. . . . The disease brings pain and, you know, nobody is really talking about that part of it. . . . So, there are things that you experience through the disease that you know—I don't know if it's just by chance or by, you know, the doctors I had, but, you know, there are things that nobody told me I might feel or experience later on.

Vickie, a sixty-year-old who received DBS for torsion dystonia and eventually had the implant removed because of cognitive and physical side effects, explained that her clinicians' focus on her tremors created a rift in their relationship. This, in her opinion, led to active harm. She pursued DBS to address an increasing difficulty in breathing, but her clinicians became determined to suppress her tremors. She told me they subjected her to a very high level of stimulation while programming her device:

> My problem was that they couldn't get my tremors under control, and I didn't want my tremors to really be a part of the whole thing. I never complained about them. I said they're not really, you know, a big issue for me. Yes, it does create lots of problems, but I'm not really targeting them. And unfortunately, they were when I didn't want that.

When I asked if she thought there was some miscommunication about her goals regarding DBS, she was emphatic:

> Absolutely not. . . . Three months after surgery, they told me they were writing up my case because it was unique, and I was the first one with dystonic tremors. So, they were after the dystonic tremors. I was not. . . . And that was not a miscommunication, because I specifically told all of them what I wanted and what I didn't care about.

The attention given to visible signifiers of difference, in part rooted in a desire to relieve stigma and incompatibilities with the built world, produced scenarios in which other, less detectable bodily experiences were overshadowed or ignored, regardless of their relative importance to the person receiving intervention.

"A Very Barbaric Situation": Embodied Experiences of Interventions

Deep brain stimulation, deployed as a metaphoric weapon against invading disability, is not the only possible intervention. As Fred stated, "It's not as if the DBS is a substitute for anything, it's an additional tool in play against the formidable enemy of the multi-symptoms of Parkinson's." Every DBS user I spoke with shared wide-ranging strategies for medical and nonmedical treatments, ranging from Botox injections to exercise classes, diet changes to medication. According to many, clinicians often present DBS as a last resort in the hierarchy of interventions because of the surgical nature of the implant. For Parkinson's disease, poor management of symptoms with medication is often a precondition for surgery. As Marty noted, when his neurologist first broached the subject, it was couched in a promise to try various medications before surgery would be considered. "He didn't jump into it, he just said, 'You would be a candidate, you know. But I think right now let's just try some different medications and see where you go with it.'"

Those medications, however, made him feel less cognitively present—which was particularly meaningful to Marty as he felt less in control of his body. John experienced compulsive gambling as a side effect of medication, although it took him several years to recognize what was happening. This left him with enormous feelings of guilt and shame. Mary, a Parkinson's blogger living in the American Southwest, shared that the mixture of her medications prior to her DBS resulted in cognitive side effects that her clinician initially misidentified, and she corrected.

Bradley expressed that his intervention options for chronic pain were DBS or narcotics, the latter of which he viewed as significantly more invasive than surgery. He told me:

> So, yeah, [DBS] was definitely a feeling of control much more so than any medication that I'd been taking, just because medication has so very specific time frames, you know, especially with narcotics, they only give you a certain amount, so if I'm having a particularly bad pain episode, there is that rationale: "Well, I

> could try to take another pill, but I only have X amount and I'll have to justify it to a doctor or I may run out."

His concerns about the surveillance that accompanies the use of narcotics were supplemented by his dismay over the disruption they caused in his life: "While I was taking all these medications, I gained fifty pounds. I was just incredibly lethargic, I mean, I felt like a zombie."

Several documents corroborated informants' perceptions of medications as significantly invasive or disruptive. One story published by a university hospital promoted DBS as an option for people whose medication regimens become unpredictable, while a children's hospital FAQ page on treating dystonia suggested that medications "do not benefit all children and can have unwanted side effects," making DBS a more attractive alternative. More commonly, however, DBS was presented as the most invasive option, with one university hospital's information sheet allowing that DBS may seem "overly aggressive and unnecessary" during the early stages of Parkinson's disease.

The above examples expose a differential understanding of risk rooted in embodiment. Medication regimens—especially those accompanied by surveillance from health care practitioners and unanticipated side effects—were perceived as more invasive and made some informants feel less in control than surgical implants. Invasiveness becomes not about transgressing the physical boundaries of the body, as assumed by nondisabled clinicians, but about social stigma, surveillance, and side effects.

The lack of information about embodied and affective experiences noted by informants in the preceding section extended into the event of receiving DBS as well. When asked what he knew about the implantation surgery prior to receiving it, John told me that although he attended a program at the hospital to learn about DBS, "I walked into it pretty blind. Pretty naive. You know, when you sit down and find out you're going to have your implant done and a hole drilled in your head, it's like, wow." As a result of this perceived lack of preparation for the physical and affective dimensions of implantation, informants reported a high degree of trauma and anxiety arising from the surgery. Descriptions of the surgery, during which the subject is typically awake to respond to lead placement, head held still by a metal cage attached to the skull, included "a very barbaric situation" (Carl) and "like throwing a bunch of walnuts in a blender with the shells on the walnuts" (John). Bradley said jokingly, "I think I probably have some minor PTSD from it," sharing that while the drilling itself was notable, he was more anxious about his involvement in ensuring proper lead placement:

> It is kind of like a bizarre thing. Because you're not quite sure what you're going to feel, you know, is it going to be painful? They're like, you know, it's a slight buzz, maybe, like I said, like a pins and needles feeling. So, there's a little bit of anxiety there of like you know waiting for it to happen and you don't know where it's going to be. Yeah, a little bit, but it wasn't an unpleasant sensation by any stretch of the imagination. And yeah, the first thought is, "Oh my god, I hope I don't mess this up." You know. I hope I don't imagine myself feeling it somewhere and they put it in the wrong spot. But it was very obvious once it started happening. It was very obvious where it was. So those fears and that anxiety quickly washed away. Yeah. So, it wasn't really too bad.

Common in all of these descriptions is a lack of awareness of what the intervention should feel like. An inattention to the bodily experience of DBS from clinicians is likely related to the fact that very few medical professionals have received DBS. This is one way in which the lived experience of disability and medical technology becomes discounted or invalidated, a topic explored in greater detail below.

Expectations of Self-Management

"I needed to lighten the load," John told me of his decision to pursue DBS after a decade with Parkinson's, "which has not been terribly lightened, but I needed to lighten the load of my lovely caregiver wife, who I owe everything to. . . . It's one of those things where you know you're a burden, but you don't know what to do about it."

Feelings of guilt and self-responsibility drove many informants' decisions to pursue deep brain stimulation, as well as their desires to take active roles in the procedure, the aftercare, and the programming of the device. Some explicitly viewed DBS as necessary for them to reemerge as productive and independent members of society, and, as such, their decisions were often couched in moralizing rhetoric. John, for example, followed up his comments quoted above by saying, "It's kind of like you die and go to heaven, and you're all upset at God and he's like, 'Well what do you mean? I gave you DBS, why didn't you try it?'" In this statement, and in the rest of the interview, it was clear that John felt doing nothing to medically intervene on his Parkinson's, when medical intervention was available and possible, was not a responsible option given his familial obligations.

Carl shared that his drive to return to work, which strongly motivated his decision to pursue DBS, was undergirded by a desire to prove himself a productive member of society:

> Currently I am looking for a job and I'm going to be studying, and hopefully I'll find something that's part-time that just helps me show parental guidance that I'm doing my best to try to function as a normal human being, if you will.

Marty's partner, Hilary, remarked about the period before Marty began telling others about his Parkinson's disease: "I mean, initially, you know, it really was very normal. We were both working. Marty was still working." The equating of "normal" with gainful employment reinscribes neoliberal ideals of individual accountability and responsibility, especially as these are linked to economic productivity, which in turn influences decisions to pursue individualized interventions for bodily nonnormativity.

For some informants, perceptions of personal accountability appeared in their judgments of others who had not pursued DBS or who had what they saw as poor outcomes from the procedure, suggesting that these outcomes often went hand in hand with poor self-management or self-advocacy. In this section, I examine the moral and social expectations that underlie decisions to pursue DBS, as well as assumptions relating the success or failure of the technology to individual agency.

"I'm Not Dissing Deep Brain Stimulation, but I Just Feel People Should Be on the Up-and-Up One Hundred Percent": Research and Risk

The reasons for pursuing DBS, or any medical intervention, are personal, variable, and contextual, and there is no unified path that all users follow prior to or after implantation. However, several common characteristics appeared throughout the informants' decision processes, including many instances of independent research, differential understandings of how and when the surgery becomes a worthwhile risk, and moralization. For some, the decision to pursue deep brain stimulation was crucially influenced by the lack of other viable options. For many, DBS seemed inevitable in the progression of care. Mary dubbed it a "quality of life decision," in part because "the reality is there's probably not going to be a magic pill ever and certainly not in our lifetime." When asked if he considered not receiving DBS, George simply stated, "I never considered not pursuing it." Marty noted that he had reached the end of his knowledge of viable alternatives before turning to DBS:

> I mean, you know, my other options were essentially like I could, I could pick up the pace of, you know, exercise in different ways you know. But you know, the reality was I didn't feel like I—I just—you know, I felt like I covered kind of most of those bases and I didn't really, you know, I researched as much as I could, like, for new things out on the horizon.

Despite the seeming inevitability of DBS in the hierarchy of increasingly complex and invasive interventions, nearly everyone I spoke with referred to an expectation and obligation to conduct a significant amount of independent research outside the clinic. The sources of information they consulted commonly included the Internet, device manufacturers, academic papers, television, and online communities. Rarely, however, were they able to meet someone with a device prior to receiving the implant.

Mary and Marty noted feeling very alienated from much of the information available about DBS, especially that coming from commercial device manufacturers. Both were diagnosed with Parkinson's at very young ages, and they did not feel represented in advertisements and user stories. Mary eventually produced her own videos and a blog sharing her experiences receiving DBS. She explained:

> I wanted someone to be able to see, because I didn't have the typical resting tremor and a lot of times in the, um, commercially produced one, the people don't look like a young onset.

> They've already got gray hair. They're sixty-five, seventy years old, and they don't look like someone who's only in their forties or thirties.

Carl and Hilary both expressed regret about not having the opportunity to do more research. Hilary, whose partner, Marty, did not experience the significant improvement to his quality of life after DBS that both had hoped for, told me she wished she had known that different types of implants were available from various manufacturers. She only learned there were multiple device manufacturers when she and Marty connected with other DBS recipients following his surgery. Carl, who experienced significant tensions with his care team as well as psychiatric institutionalization following the surgery, regretted not considering additional hospitals before he received treatment. He said:

> My best advice is for anybody that wants to get deep brain stimulation is to really do your research with the hospitals that are available in your area or what your insurance can cover, and really extensively take your time with the neurologist and really heavily discuss everything from A to Z, meaning side effects that people have experienced during the surgery, such as infection, which has been a lot of the bigger issues, a lot of people are getting infections after the surgery, and also sharing any other side effects that people have been experiencing later down the road from deep brain stimulation so that they know what they are getting into. And that's my best, final statement to say about deep brain stimulation. I'm not dissing deep brain stimulation, but I just feel people should be on the up-and-up one hundred percent.

The prevalence of independent research and risk analysis among informants may be linked in important ways to the sense of personal responsibility many felt when pursuing DBS. This feeling of responsibility extended not only to receiving the implant itself but also to being informed users. It may reveal informants' sense that they received inadequate information in the clinic. Given the experiences summarized above, in which people felt underprepared both for their conditions and for DBS, it is perhaps unsurprising that they felt the need to seek information outside the clinic.

The decision to pursue DBS was also influenced by the individual's own contextual and personal risk calculus. Fred, who had originally planned to have DBS in the summer of 2014, pushed the date up by about six months when he felt the benefits had started to outweigh the risks: "The reason I made that decision that I had to do it now was it's not going to get any better if I wait. If I wait six months, it's not getting any better. I'll be in worse shape if anything, because I can't exercise." For Marty, the decision was made after one specific incident where he felt himself "run out of gas" during an exercise class, which indicated for him that the risks of surgery were now more in balance with the possible benefits. For more than half of informants, the risk calculus was influenced by the closing time window articulated by their clinicians, whether that was an age cutoff or other criteria. "There's a window of opportunity there," as Mary said, "where you get to the point where you're not eligible anymore." This time crunch heavily factored in the decision-making process for some people, while others were more motivated by their perceived decline in function.

For Vickie, in retrospect the risk of the implant was ultimately not worth the benefits. Even as she experienced some improvements in her quality of life, the cognitive effects she experienced postimplant counteracted any potential benefits, leading to her eventually turning off the device and seeking its removal. She warned others to develop their own risk analysis carefully:

> So, I mean, it was kind of nice having the relief, a little bit of relief, but not at the expense of me being totally out of it. And not at the expense of my mind or my, you know, my brain. . . . I don't feel it was worth it and I would not do it again. And I would not advise anyone to do it without being fully informed, and they do not fully inform you.

Upon receiving DBS, many informants found themselves in new roles, serving as resources for other potential DBS users, helping them to fill the knowledge gaps they themselves had encountered. Many volunteered to speak to other potential DBS users, worked to educate clinicians, or shared their experiences in online and in-person support groups. Mary educated medical students so that people with DBS admitted to hospitals would not have to. Bradley spoke to other people who had strokes to advocate for the use of DBS during recovery. He stated:

> I think honestly one of the coolest things that come from all of this is that I get to be—become an advocate for it and that's one of the things that I've honestly tried to do the most since having the stroke and especially since having the surgery and having the DBS and everything is just trying to reach out to other people that are going through this in any way.

John began to share his experiences with DBS with his Parkinson's support group because he realized he was not receiving the support he needed for the issues he brought to the sessions, and he planned to stop attending. "But then I started looking a little different," he said. "How can I help these people? I need to give a little bit. Open my heart. Give a little bit. Help try to bring these guys up to speed." This statement is embedded with judgment about the kinds of people who attended the support group. John viewed them not as peers with whom he could empathize but as people in need of assistance that he saw himself as capable of providing. This reframing allowed him to continue attending, albeit with altered expectations.

Themes of DBS users' altruism toward others who may seek treatment also featured in several human interest and patient success stories produced by hospital systems. In one such story, published by a university hospital, the person who received DBS was described as "a familiar face at [university hospital], where she serves as a cheerleader for DBS and the [university's] efforts to help Parkinson's patients live better lives." The article reported that she volunteered to speak to both medical students and potential DBS users, noting "you have to have that kind of support" when deciding to pursue DBS. As echoed in the interviews, this example displays users identifying a gap in support, whether that be in clinician education or in the communities receiving DBS, and feeling compelled to fill it with their own knowledge, often pro bono. Informants and documentation praised the (almost universally uncompensated) labor of DBS users as vital to the DBS journey, even as users experienced invalidation in clinical interactions. This tension exemplifies one facet of the double bind of responsibility and passivity confronting DBS users.

"Work Hard and Be a Good Person": Moralizing DBS

John told me that he felt an obligation to pursue DBS in order to "be a better person" for his family, especially his wife, who was also his current caregiver. He said:

> It's just a mindset. Get your shit together, John. Quit feeling sorry for yourself. What are you doing? You know? You have to take care of [indecipherable] yourself. You know? It's kind of like my children—I don't want them thinking, "Why isn't Dad doing something? He's just sitting there."

Rachel, John's wife, followed up by saying, "John is, and always has been, just very positive, very appreciative, very helpful. He doesn't feel sorry for himself."

His decision to pursue DBS was couched in a morality lesson for his children about responsibility and familial obligation, which ascribed a value judgment not only to himself but also to others who do or do not pursue intervention. This was reinforced by several anecdotes he shared about acquaintances with Parkinson's. One friend had recently been institutionalized after threatening his wife. Another's wife had told him she would no longer be his caregiver. Each of these cautionary stories ended with an assertion that people with Parkinson's need to "share the burden" of management and "just keep your mouth shut and be a good person. Work hard and be a good person." One university hospital released an informational sheet on facts and myths about Parkinson's disease that echoed John's sentiment, stating flatly, "This 'it is what it is; there's nothing I can do to help myself' myth is counterproductive." Such pronouncements connote an assumption that many people with Parkinson's are not experiencing good quality of life owing to an unwillingness to take responsibility for their own well-being.

Occasionally, these feelings among informants manifested in judgment of others for either not pursuing DBS or experiencing negative outcomes. As Mary noted, "If you don't do self-management, you're not going to have a good outcome." This view was further defined by a delineation of requirements for technical expertise as a DBS recipient. Mary continued, "In fact I have often even said if you couldn't program your VCR you probably have no business getting DBS unless you're going to take some responsibility for—be your own advocate."

Through such statements, a picture of a "worthy" DBS user emerged: outspoken, educated, self-motivated, and grateful. For Lynn, receiving DBS allowed her to make downward social comparisons against those with similar disabilities who have not been implanted. "I think that I'm kind of a step ahead of everybody else because I've had DBS," she said. "Most people have not had it. I'm shocked. . . . Nobody has DBS. I think, 'Why not? Look at you.'"

In addition to the moralization of the decision to pursue implantation itself, both positive and negative outcomes following implantation were accompanied by feelings of responsibility, perceived as either success or failure to manage one's body and one's clinical relationships properly. Barry, Mary's husband, expressed pride in Mary's relationship with her clinicians and the device manufacturers, which he saw as enabling an enhanced level of care: "It's because of the advocacy work that she does that she gets a special bond. That's what it is. She earns it. I shouldn't say she's lucky. She earns it." This statement, through its framing, suggests that the extra work Mary put into developing relationships, including teaching medical students and developing a telemedicine service in her area, entitled her to receive better care than someone who was simply the recipient of medical services. Mary supported this perspective, noting, "Their [the neurologist and neurosurgeon's] job is to fix the problem in your brain. It's your job to learn everything else."

Conversely, Carl linked his bad experiences with DBS to his taking action outside his role as passive recipient of technology, as described in the opening of this chapter. From his perspective, by stepping into a more active role and using his patient remote to adjust his stimulation levels, he took on authority that belonged to his clinician. In this framing, his auditory hallucinations were punishment for that transgression. He was expected, as a medical technology user, to be responsible, but he was disallowed from being authoritative, a subject I take up more explicitly in the following section.

This perspective directly contradicts many of the documents analyzed for this case, which often couched themes of self-responsibility in a rhetoric of empowerment. For example, an informational news story published by a university hospital closed by quoting a neurosurgeon who advised, "It's up to the patients to decide whether the problems are significant enough to take the small but present risks of the procedure in order to achieve those results." Such a statement is outwardly empowering, yet it simultaneously shifts the onus of responsibility away from the clinicians and onto the individual to do the complicated risk calculus articulated by informants above.

Authority and Invalidation

Carl's experience of invalidation and institutionalization, described at this chapter's opening, exemplifies the epistemic invalidation shared by many informants who received DBS. From a lack of attention to embodiment to the seeming dismissal of mental health as linked to neurological health, for most, the bodymind was not interpreted as a source of expertise in clinical settings, despite clear stated value in experiential knowledge outside these settings. Epistemic invalidation often occurred even prior to clinical diagnosis, and experiential but difficult-to-quantify symptoms were often dismissed. Mary and Fred, for example, both shared that their initial diagnoses of Parkinson's were delayed by several years when the symptoms they reported to clinicians were dismissed out of hand. Invalidation was often paired with an assertion of medical authority as credible and trustworthy, an argument raised in much of the documentation as well. This perception of medical authority appeared throughout the interviews, with several informants undermining their own experiential knowledge in favor of medical expertise. In many instances, invalidation occurred specifically when the line between the neurological and the psychological was blurred, such as in the attribution of mental health issues to an implant for movement disorders. In some cases, when self-knowledge was invalidated by medical authorities, informants turned to informal user or patient communities, such as support groups and online forums, for validation and resources. In this section, I examine the social economies that establish clinicians as authorities on embodiment in DBS implantation, tracing the perceived markers of trust and credibility among clinicians as well as the importance of experiential knowledge in day-to-day life with DBS. I close by interrogating the invalidation experienced by recipients of DBS when their perceptions come into conflict with clinical authority.

"Thank You for Trusting Us with Your Care": Establishing Medical Authority

The authority of clinicians, including neurosurgeons, neurologists, primary care physicians, and other medical professionals, was articulated by informants in terms of credibility-building practices to establish trust as well as stable and open communication. When Marty was deciding to pursue DBS, these were both crucial factors. "Okay, if I'm going to do this . . . this is a good surgeon," he said. "He's got a good reputation, you know. I felt like he was honest with me and answered the questions." Trust in clinicians performing DBS was established through a series of factors, including the clinician's or clinic's status or reputation, preestablished relationships, and the scientific or technical naming, classification, and/or visualization of the person's condition.

Marty, who expressed some trepidation prior to receiving DBS and some doubts that it had been effective at the time of his interview, stated that the procedure must have some value, or the doctors he received it from would not have suggested it:

> You know, I guess one thing in my brain is I will tell myself that I find it hard to believe that, you know, two doctors, both with very good reputations, you know, they're both like the big man on campus in the area. I find it hard to believe that the two of them would conspire to trick all these people into having brain surgery that isn't actually doing anything. You know, I know that sounds kind of crude and a stupid way of thinking, but in reality, like, I would hate to think that two people would be that money driven or that ego driven to believe or project that it does more than it does. I mean, do they sell it? Do they encourage people to do it? Probably. I'm sure they do. I'm sure they believe in it, you know. And I know it's not going to have the same effect on every single person. Clearly. But you know, I believe, I believe to some degree that it has to work [that] way.

He ultimately decided to trust his clinicians because he believed they could not maintain their high status and reputation if they were untrustworthy. This statement, however, was made in retrospect, and it signaled some of the doubt he felt afterward when he did not achieve the outcomes he was expecting. He acknowledged the marketing aspect of DBS, but ultimately reaffirmed that he trusted his clinicians' intentions.

For others, like Vickie, trust came from long-standing relationships with their care teams. When I asked Vickie whether she had felt any concerns prior to surgery about cognitive side effects like what she eventually experienced, she noted:

> I can't really say that I felt suspicious. I asked my doctor about [cognitive side effects]. He said definitely there will be none. And I'd gone there for twenty-five years, so I was inclined to believe him. . . . I actually was very relaxed during surgery. I believed them, that was the only place I trusted. They were the ones who first diagnosed me.

While initially Vickie was confident in her care team because of the long-term relationship, her trust eventually eroded as a result of mismatched priorities and a perceived power imbalance. She felt that her clinician was focusing all his attention on her tremors and ignoring both the symptom she was most concerned about (difficulty breathing) and the side effects she was experiencing postimplant, and she became resentful. She told me: "His ego was in the way. It was like he had to somehow conquer my brain. And conquer these tremors and make them go away." Clinical authority quickly shifted from being a source of comfort to being a source of resentment when authority to make decisions on the DBS user's behalf became a form of control.

As detailed in previous sections, as disability comes to be defined as a lack of bodily control, DBS is configured as a method of reestablishing order. This is achieved not only through the use of the device itself, which for some enables control of symptoms they deem to be interfering with their quality of life, but also through an acquisition of scientific and medical knowledge about the body mind. Visualization and measurement techniques allowed informants to accumulate medical and scientific knowledge about their bodies, which in turn bolstered the credibility of their clinicians. Bradley noted, for example, that he was reassured when his clinician "actually showed me the exact spot on my brain that was literally the size of a pin tip that was causing all of these problems and had all of this data." He continued: "Seeing the postsurgery or postimplant MRI and seeing exactly where it's placed compared to [where] the actual specific damaged spot was in the brain" was "eye-opening" and "kind of comforting, knowing that I have control over it." The identification of a physiological locus of his pain, which previously felt unknowable, factored into his understanding of control. His clinician established credibility through his seeming abundance of data, concretizing the ambiguous nature of Bradley's pain through visualization and technical explanations.

Documentation also linked knowledge acquisition to control. A brochure from a university hospital's movement disorder clinic made this connection most explicitly by inviting patients to attend conferences, declaring, "When it comes to the fight against Parkinson's disease, knowledge is power." Such statements not only reiterate the perceived combative relationship between disabled bodyminds and the people who occupy them but also emphasize that medical knowledge is a crucial weapon in that battle. Resonating with the elements of clinical interactions that established clinical authority for informants, the majority of documents also engaged in credibility-building discourses by providing information about clinicians' credentials, hospital rankings, and other elements to reaffirm the expertise and credibility of clinicians and hospitals and their ability to perform successful DBS intervention. Often, these credibility statements included information about the historical or unique role the hospital or an affiliated clinician played in DBS research and development. For example, a neurological center framed its informational page about DBS by saying that its "neurosurgeons and neurologists were involved in early clinical trials of the therapy and have developed expertise that is hard to find in this emerging field." Additionally, many materials included statistics and technical explanations as strategies for building trust and credibility.

Methods of communication were also key to either bolstering or eroding clinical authority during surgery and programming. Fred and Nora found the holistic communication they received from social workers, nurses, the neurosurgeon, the neurologist, and representatives of the device manufacturer was crucial to their perception of the procedure and outcomes. For them and several others, the willingness of the care team to openly discuss the possible negative outcomes cemented their trust in clinical authority, in part because it was an admission of uncertainty. As Nora said, these conversations helped Fred with the process of "trying to balance all that" as he made the decision to pursue DBS. Communication also became key for the surgery process itself. Bradley said that his clinician's talking through all the steps of the surgery aloud, which he was doing for the benefit of a medical student in the room, had a calming effect for him. Further, "he was constantly checking on me, and it was just so reassuring laying out all the steps."

Communication was sometimes perceived as a one-way channel, however, to the frustration of several informants. Mary, who herself had been engaged in education and advocacy projects, bluntly noted, "I believe as I said it would be nice if you could get several Parkinson's folks to speak to a lot of doctors. But the reality is that it's doctors speaking to folks with Parkinson's." This statement suggests a rigidity to this relationship, a point both Mary and her husband, Barry, reiterated frequently throughout their interview. As Barry commented when Mary suggested she would like to see a roomful of clinicians listening to a panel of people with Parkinson's: "You couldn't arrange that. [Clinicians] wouldn't come." In their estimation, clinicians do not have the time or interest to learn from users, which further contributes to the shifting of the onus of responsibility onto users to be self-motivated and self-responsible. That onus, as alluded to by several informants, includes educating physicians who are not experts on DBS. John noted he was the first person with DBS that his general practitioner had ever encountered, forcing John into an educator role. He told me, "This is the curve, you know? And so when I go in and talk to him, I tell him—I enlighten him a bit every time I can." His embodied and experiential knowledge suddenly became an asset in this situation, and his responsibility for his care took on an additional dimension.

As in the interviews, the importance of clinical communication was highlighted in the documentation, often to build trust in clinicians and establish user autonomy and empowerment. One health service system made the following recommendation on its informational page: "You and your neurologist should discuss the role of DBS in your long-term treatment plan early after your diagnosis with Parkinson's disease." With its suggestion of opportunities for collaborative decision-making, this statement is embedded with assumptions about bidirectional communication, user engagement, shared priorities, and transparency—assumptions that were not reflected in informants' stories. Another document took clinical trust as a given, stating simply at the top of its DBS informational page, "Thank you for trusting us with your care."

"We're Not a Patient, We're Not a Client, We're a Person": Embodied Expertise and Invalidation

Informants expressed the value of their embodied and experiential knowledge in their day-to-day care practices, the priorities they set for their treatment plans, and their interactions with both clinicians and other users. The knowledge that arises from occupying a nonnormative bodymind is essential and underrecognized in clinical settings, in part because of the relegation of the patient to a one-dimensional, passive role. As Fred asserted, "We're not a patient, we're not a client, we're a person." He continued by sharing the advice he provides whenever he speaks about disability with nondisabled people: "When you ask somebody with Parkinson's—or other disorders, other disabilities as well—If they say they're okay, well, believe them. So, if the person says they're all right, believe them. That's one thing you need to do." He and others expressed that there is no one who knows more about themselves than they do, and yet that knowledge is constantly dismissed or invalidated in public and clinical settings.

Mary argued that as a person with Parkinson's, she knows much more about the condition than her clinicians, just by virtue of the time she spends thinking about it. "So actually, it will end up being fifteen months between appointments and I'll probably have a half hour appointment with [the neurologist]," she said, "but the rest of those bazillion hours and minutes, guess who manages my Parkinson's? Me."

Just as John's knowledge about DBS became an important element of his care with his general practitioner, several informants argued that more clinician attentiveness to what they know could transform their care. For example, as discussed in the Introduction, Mary noted that the type of pulse generator she had implanted in her chest has a squared edge. This shape makes it impossible for her to shave her armpits, a drawback that affects her quality of life and self-image. She also mentioned a patient remote in development that was operated by touch screen rather than analog buttons. While this design might seem more convenient to non-users, Mary pointed out that people with dexterity limitations—which can be caused by many of the conditions for which DBS is recommended—are often not able to operate touch screens effectively, so the remote would be useless to them. Her husband, Barry, observed that "if they had talked to the patient first, they would've pointed that out right away. You're going in the wrong direction here." He argued that "people with Parkinson's should be the ones who are designing these things."

Very few documents addressed the experiential knowledge of DBS users, with the exception of those that reinforced the need for users to serve as educators for nonexperts such as emergency room attendants and general practitioners. In the documents examined, there were no suggestions of or allusions to the incorporation of DBS user input into the design and implementation of DBS. Additionally, despite informants' articulated understanding of the value of their embodied and experiential expertise, the majority experienced invalidation of their experiences, knowledge, and personhood from their clinicians. This was particularly prevalent when their experiences of DBS blurred the lines between the neurological and the psychological. Not only was their self-knowledge delegitimated, but in the process, the users were recast as passive or helpless—as patients, rather than people.

As discussed above, when their embodied experience was invalidated by clinicians, some informants turned to informal patient communities for validation and resources. For example, when Mary began experiencing depression and suicidal thoughts and suspected that her DBS was a contributing factor, she was rebuffed by several clinicians before eventually having her experience corroborated by a DBS recipient online:

> I reached out to the local doctor and said, "Is there any chance my settings can be causing my depression?" No. And I went to the movement disorder specialist in [city], "Is there any chance that my settings could be causing my depression?" No. And all they want to do is put me on antidepressants, which just made me feel even worse. . . . So then I reached out to my online community via Facebook, and I said, "Is there any chance that my settings can cause depression?" And within minutes I got a reply back . . . so she actually called me and said yes.

Mary, through her connection with another DBS user who had been part of a clinical trial interrogating the effects of DBS on mood, was able to find support to reprogram her device. Mary's experience, which echoes the denials Carl encountered when experiencing psychiatric symptoms following his implantation, reveals a pattern in which recipients of DBS, rather than having their mental health treated as linked to (and in fact inseparable from) their neurological and physical health, had their psychological symptoms dismissed or treated with condescension or blame.

Marty noted clinical dismissal of his increasingly high anxiety, despite the fact that he felt it was exacerbated by poor clinical communication:

> That's an excuse to say, "Well, the reason why you're acting this way is because you just, you just get too anxious about what setting you should be on." And that's not really, that's not why—I'm anxious or I'm getting anxious because, you know, you're not telling me the right information or, you know, I can't sleep and you're giving me this kind of medication [anxiolytics] instead of a medication that will help me sleep.

George shared experiencing anxiety after receiving DBS as well, but admitted his uncertainty as to its source, noting, "I don't know if there is a connection or if perhaps it is just age-related."

Overall, these experiences of epistemic invalidation exemplify a forced distinction between the neurological and the psychological—the brain versus the mind—in the clinic. Additionally, the privileging of clinical or medical authority over self-knowledge, which has been demonstrated throughout this chapter, creates scenarios in which users look for validation from their clinicians and experience distress when they do not receive it. Through these examples, it is clear that epistemic invalidation has significant impacts on DBS users, and that it is especially prevalent when users bring forward psychological, affective, or psychiatric concerns.

In contrast to some of the informants' experiences of epistemic invalidation around psychological or affective issues following DBS, several of the materials produced by hospital systems acknowledged the potential of DBS to affect mood or personality. One hospital system listed among the potential side effects of DBS "changes in personality, behavior, memory, thinking or language skills (including confusion)," and another stated that "DBS does not help improve the cognitive and emotional symptoms of Parkinson's disease, such as depression or memory loss. In fact, it can make these symptoms worse." The disconnect between the written communications and the in situ experiences of the people interviewed in this study raises concerns about mixed messages and variable standards of care.

Self-Governance and Clinical Authority with Deep Brain Stimulation

In this chapter, I have grappled with the tensions around knowledge, power, and responsibility that characterize users' experiences of deep brain stimulation. These tensions fall into two broad categories: those related to how the body (and biomedical intervention) is interpreted and made meaningful, and those related to the moralization of technological intervention and self-governance. Before concluding, I also discuss gender as a particularly meaningful analytical framework for grappling with the neoliberal expectations of individual productivity and disabled bodyminds.

Transgressing the Body

Normative understandings of the bodymind permeate experiences of choosing and using DBS. As Jonathan Mathers and colleagues found in their exploration of the use of DBS for Parkinson's disease, the choice to receive deep brain stimulation is often characterized by hope for a return to normality, where "normality" means a predisabled state.[15] As shown in this chapter, disability is signified by both loss of agency over one's body and loss of social control through visual markers of difference such as tremors. Previous qualitative literature on experiences of deep brain stimulation (usually relating to Parkinson's) also affirms the stigma of visual difference through tremor as a primary motivator for pursuing DBS, despite the fact that, as Gun-Marie Hariz, Patricia Limousin, and Katarina Hamberg write, "tremor is not considered as the [Parkinson's] symptom that contributes most to disability or impacts most on quality of life."[16] This contradiction is meaningful: Despite ample qualitative research emphasizing social stigma as central to decisions to pursue DBS, in the clinic, disability and quality of life are defined much more narrowly, and more physiologically.

An additional contradiction further muddies the place of tremor and other observable signifiers of difference for people pursuing DBS. As explored above, an overemphasis on tremor leads to the invisibilization of other aspects of disease progression, exemplified by Marty's recollection of never having been told by a physician that Parkinson's disease can be physically painful. Further, any operationalization of disability that focuses solely on reshaping the bodymind fails to attend to the social, attitudinal, and infrastructural ableism that led Marty to query, "Why is there nowhere for me to sit down?" Imagining disability as an entanglement of the social and the embodied can open up new pathways for intervention, as opposed to the assumed inevitability of DBS as expressed by many in this case.

Additionally, norms around the perceived value of the whole and unviolated bodymind configure DBS as a "last resort" technology, as found both in this chapter and in previous research, obscuring the ways in which seemingly less invasive interventions may in fact be more disruptive to everyday life. Many medical professionals consider the surgical implantation of a deep brain stimulator to be significantly more invasive than medication regimens because of the transgression of the physical boundaries of the body through surgery. People receiving the procedure, however, have asserted the invasiveness of medications, whether through their physical side effects, such as involuntary movements caused by the commonly used Parkinson's medication levodopa, or through the surveillance by medical professionals necessary for their use. For these users, surgery, despite its "transgressive" nature, was less worrisome both because their disabled bodyminds were already subject to invasive medical procedures in the course of regular care and because surgery signaled the introduction of a system that they could control. Daniel Alfonso and colleagues found something similar, reporting that while the majority of people with Parkinson's surveyed in their study would consider medication changes before DBS, many did not consider DBS to be a "last resort."[17] As Bradley pointed out when he recounted being offered either narcotics or surgery: "But when you look at narcotics, it's invasive in a much more perverse way. You know, it's not, your body's not being cut open, but it's so invasive in your life in so many other facets. So, I think we're taking a very simplistic look at it when it's obviously much bigger." This "life invasiveness" again signals the need to consider holistic approaches that take into account the impacts of medical interventions on people's lives, not just on their symptoms.

Bodily Responsibility under Neoliberal Conditions

The pressures of neoliberal ableism and modernity bear on disabled bodyminds in unique ways, as has been evidenced in this chapter.[18] Neoliberal values of independence and autonomy contributed to many informants' perceptions of themselves and their responsibility to manage their bodyminds in specific ways. Interventions on nonnormative bodyminds—such as medical interventions—are individualized and privatized but are understood as being for the public good. For informants, values including independence, autonomy, and a return to financial productivity at times drove the decision to receive an implant and consequently contributed to feelings of disappointment, guilt, and shame if these goals proved unattainable. Given the entanglement of social and technological progress in American culture, and the increasing reliance on technoscience that characterizes the era of biomedicalization, fulfilling one's responsibilities toward becoming self-governing, autonomous, and productive means embracing technological intervention.[19] As adoption of technological interventions becomes a moral imperative, personal decisions about one's health and body become decisions for the public good. Health, illness, and disability are increasingly entwined with the processes and expectations of good citizenship. For some, like Carl, this meant attempting to return to the workforce. While discourse around the adoption of DBS is shot through with the rhetoric of choice and empowerment, these social and political pressures—amplified by structural ableism—demand personal responsibility.

This looming pressure to approximate the idealized bodymind is what Robert McRuer calls "compulsory able-bodiedness." Inspired by Adrienne Rich's 1980 essay on "compulsory heterosexuality," McRuer articulates a culture in which normative (ideal) bodies are naturalized as both an expected default and the moral obligation.[20] In such a system, one is confronted constantly with the seeming choice of whether or not to augment and intervene on one's nonnormative bodymind, but McRuer argues that in reality, there is no choice but to intervene. Under a regime of compulsory able-bodiedness,

> able-bodied identities, able-bodied perspectives are preferable and what we all, collectively, are aiming for. A system of compulsory able-bodiedness repeatedly demands that people with disabilities embody for others an affirmative answer to the unspoken question, Yes, but in the end, wouldn't you rather be more like me?[21]

Compulsory able-bodiedness, therefore, is tightly coupled with "questions of cure, loss, and disavowal," according to Alison Kafer.[22] These pressures to return to a predisabled idealized state through DBS were felt acutely by nearly every user I spoke with. The notable exception was Vickie, who was born with her disability, and who expressed that her tremors—which visibly marked her nonnormativity—were not a concern to her.

Intervening on Disabled Masculinities

While no comprehensive data are available on the demographics of DBS usage, we know that in the United States those who are most likely to receive DBS for Parkinson's disease are cisgender men, white, privately insured, and financially well-off.[23] The majority of DBS users I spoke with were white, cisgender men, many of whom evoked gender and gendered expectations as significant in their experience of disability and DBS. Resonating with previous work on masculinity and acquired disability, disability's challenge to masculinity proved a crucial phenomenon through which to interpret informants' experiences.[24] As Helen Meekosha writes, "The image of disability may be intensified by gender—for women a sense of intensified passivity and helplessness, for men a corrupted masculinity generated by enforced dependence."[25] "Masculinity" here does not refer to some innate or biological characteristic, but to hegemonic masculinity, or the set of practices that legitimate male dominance and control.[26] In Western culture, this masculinity is typified by de facto heterosexuality, competition, economic success in a capitalist market, and suppression of vulnerability. Disability confronts hegemonic masculinity on a collective level by producing alternative masculine imaginaries, and—when disability is acquired, as is the case with many of the conditions intervened on by DBS—on an individual level as the person grapples with their fluid social standing.

Common among the male-identifying informants in this case were expressions of hope for reclaiming hegemonic masculinity through technological intervention. For example, Carl spoke openly about the shame and disappointment that came with realizing that he would not be able to return to work after he received his DBS. He pointed to moving back in with his parents as a particularly demoralizing moment that spurred him to start making, in his words, "more healthy decisions" because "I'm a middle-aged man now living at home, so it makes you wake up, if you will." He particularly advocated for a type of masculine stoicism for himself and others experiencing similar circumstances, noting that it is best to be a "silent warrior" and to "stop pointing fingers and just deal with it and be a man. Sorry, I should say, I don't want to sound sexist, be a strong person. A person with strength." John spoke about his desire to relieve the caregiving burden he felt his disability imposed, sharing that he chose to pursue DBS to "be of service to my family, to my wife." His desire to regain his independence and to provide for his family, thus reclaiming his masculinity, directly influenced his decision to pursue medical technology.

Ultimately, contests of authority, neoliberal responsibility, and the perceived validity of knowledge over disability animate discourses and interactions around deep brain stimulation. While users are expected to independently research and self-calculate acceptable risks associated with interventions (risks that, in the case of DBS, are judged directly in relation to how distressing preoperative symptoms are),[27] ultimate authority over disabled bodyminds is very much ceded to clinicians. The epistemic authority of medicine over disability, which results in invalidation—as many informants experienced when their bodyminds came into conflict with the medical establishment—demands the simultaneous suppression of other ways of knowing and being. For example, underwritten by the perceived distinction between mind and body, explicit and implicit boundaries between the neurological and the psychological are drawn in the clinic, leading to epistemic invalidation for those who blur the boundaries. Marty, Carl, and Mary all recalled periods of mental distress following their DBS surgeries, ranging from anxiety to suicidal ideation to hallucinations, and all had these experiences dismissed by clinicians as unrelated to their neurology. Disability studies scholars have long argued against the false division between mind and body, pushing against the entrenchment of the Cartesian dualism that characterizes much of Western medicine and social practices.[28]

Langdon Winner suggests that technologies must be judged not only for "their contributions to efficiency and productivity," which in this case would consist of the management of unruly disabled bodyminds, but also for "the ways in which they embody specific forms of power and authority."[29] Key to the management of the neoliberal subject is the ability to make all individuals commensurable. In other words, it is necessary to take the idiosyncratic and fit it into a category that can be understood and intervened upon. The medicalization of certain phenomena enables this type of categorizing and flattening. As a result, the kinds of knowledge that allow for this commensuration become authoritative. As discussed above, medical authority takes precedence over embodied and experiential expertise, so disabled individuals lose credibility to speak on their own bodyminds. With this loss of credibility comes also a loss of agency to choose for oneself in social and medical interactions. The pressures of neoliberalism complicate this process, producing a double bind in which individuals are held personally accountable for managing their nonnormative bodies—where personal accountability means pursuing individualized, privatized medical intervention—while at the same time their knowledge about their bodies is questioned, ignored, or invalidated. The following chapter, which explores do-it-yourself medical technologies in type 1 diabetes communities, presents a rebuttal to this systemic invalidation through the coherence of user communities developing and using technology apart from medical authority.

« 4 »

Reimagining Agency with Do-It-Yourself Artificial Pancreas Systems

When Erica was in high school, she "just completely stopped doing diabetes." Diagnosed with type 1 diabetes as a toddler, she had been giving herself insulin shots independently since she was ten years old. "And because I'd been diabetic for so long in the health care system," she told me, "everyone assumes that I know everything already." She recalled one endocrinologist giving her "intricate concepts about insulin and dosing" that she didn't understand, when what she needed was practical advice to build a "foundation of good care." Without knowledge and with the expectation that she, as a teenager, was solely responsible for her daily management, Erica floundered. She lied to her parents about her blood sugar and failed to give herself insulin regularly. "I still don't understand how I'm like here and breathing. I was so negligent."

As she got older, Erica decided she wanted to learn more about her body. She began to teach herself. She inhaled all the information about diabetes she could find, consulting her local library, diabetes organizations, and other people with T1D. She became very involved in T1D organizations, and she began to hear about do-it-yourself artificial pancreas systems, which usurp preexisting diabetes technologies for more customized, less intensive daily management. At first, Erica was unsure about DIY. She described her hesitance: "What I thought was I'd be entering into this kind of weird, almost like dark web medical device hackers on the Internet who I don't know and maybe it's kind of seedy." Besides, she had been managing her diabetes well in her early adulthood and did not feel that she needed to explore options outside her current management strategies. But as more of her friends started looking into DIY, she became more curious. Soon, on a stop during a cycling trip, she found herself in the home of a prominent DIYer. Here, Erica began to see a different DIY community than she had imagined. After extending a warm greeting, the DIYer mentioned that she had just spoken to their mutual friend and passed on a message of love to Erica. "And I just started crying," Erica said. "Oh, okay, there's no scary hacker lady here. This woman was just talking to my friend. And I just started bawling. I'd had a long day cycling and it was nice to know that someone cared for me." Six hours later, Erica had all of her tech set up to start using her own artificial pancreas system.

In this chapter, I examine the histories and experiences of users of DIY artificial pancreas systems to grapple with the relationship between the technification of medicine for chronic illness and feelings of individual responsibility and agency. The DIYers I spoke with identified with a strong ethos of self-responsibility in response to a medical establishment that failed to meet their needs or take their desires into account. Embodiment and experience, which are often dismissed in the clinic, are taken as credible markers of expertise among DIYAPS users. Further, an emphasis on decentralization, transparency, and collaboration in DIY spaces creates conditions for producing and sharing knowledge that are different from those found in traditional medical professional–patient relationships. I draw on interviews with sixteen informants, ten pursuing DIY artificial pancreas systems for themselves and six acting as guardians for children using DIY systems, as well as documentation produced by DIY communities, blogs, and regulators.[1] Unlike much of the documentation explored in the cases of prenatal genetic testing and deep brain stimulation, the majority of the material I analyzed was written by users themselves, including some informants. I articulate three key knowledge transgressions foundational to the emergence and flourishing of DIYAPS: first, the abandonment of the curative promise that enables professionals and traditional experts to retain control; second, the rearticulation of risk and responsibility informed by embodiment; and third, the transformation of diabetes from a hyperindividualized experience to a communal one. I conclude the chapter with a closer analysis of the meaning and consequences of these transgressions, namely, the generative alternatives made possible by the formation of a space built on embodied and experiential knowledge.

Do-It-Yourself, Together

In 2013, Dana Lewis had a problem. As she recounted in a 2018 TEDx talk, she had been living with T1D for most of her life, but the technologies she relied on were failing her. In particular, the continuous glucose monitor that alerted her when her blood sugar was dangerously high or low did not have an alarm loud enough to wake her up. Without an adequate alarm, she was not able to compensate for overnight blood sugar fluctuations, which could lead to coma or death. After receiving a noncommittal response from the manufacturer of her CGM, Lewis took matters into her own hands. With the assistance of code from John Costik, the parent of a child with T1D who had figured out how to access his child's CGM data remotely, Lewis was able to upload her CGM data from her receiver to her computer, where she could control the alarm volume more easily. But Lewis did not stop there. Combining the newly accessible data with information about insulin dosing and food intake, she and others in the T1D community were able to develop predictive algorithms that provided recommendations based on forecast blood glucose levels. A little over one year later, working with Ben West and Scott Leibrand, Lewis "closed the loop" when she figured out how to use the algorithm they had created to control her insulin dosing through an insulin pump. Thus, the first do-it-yourself artificial pancreas system was born.[2] According to OpenAPS, a community aiming to make safe and effective APS technology available through open-source projects and community collaboration, as of March 2024, there were more than 3,200 DIY closed-loop users around the world, with more than 100 million "loop hours."[3]

Both traditional and user-led research communities are increasingly interested in the clinical outcomes related to DIYAPS. A 2018 retrospective study conducted by OpenAPS community members in the United States found that, for the twenty users surveyed, blood glucose, A1C, and glucose time in range all improved through the use of OpenAPS.[4] Similarly, that same year, a study in Italy with thirty participants showed statistically significant changes in A1C and time in hypoglycemia through the use of OpenAPS.[5] Research conducted in South Korea with twenty children also showed significant benefits from OpenAPS, including decreased A1C, increased time in range, and decreased time in hypo- or hyperglycemia.[6] Beyond clinical markers of disease management, a self-reported survey produced by the OpenAPS community reported better quality of life through "increased time in range, uninterrupted sleep, and peace of mind."[7] The entirety of the DIYAPS community is a very small fraction of the estimated nine million people living with T1D globally, however, and one that some argue is a subset of people with diabetes who are especially tech savvy or engaged in their management.[8] Since DIYAPS hit the scene, several commercially available hybrid loop systems have come to market in both the United States and Europe. These devices have received some criticism for a lack of customizability in comparison with DIY options, and preliminary research suggests high abandonment rates in situ.[9] Several other closed-loop or automated insulin delivery systems are currently in development, some based on DIY algorithms and systems. For example, Tidepool Loop, an automated dosing application based on DIY algorithms, received FDA clearance in 2023.[10]

From Cure to Quality of Life

When I spoke to Gary, a man in his thirties living in the Midwest, he had been living with T1D for just two years. Diagnosed as an adult, he was immediately suspicious of a medical establishment that was populated primarily by people without diabetes and that held expectations for outcomes that were difficult to achieve using current clinical best practices. He expressed exasperation at the blame that clinicians place on people with T1D, noting that current on-label treatments—even when people with T1D can access them and have support from knowledgeable clinicians—make it nearly impossible for users to achieve optimum results. "There's a lot of blaming patients for not getting desirable results," he said. "And right now if you are sticking to the book, I don't think it's possible to get anywhere near the desirable temp 7 percent [A1C] target that all the professional associations want."

For people without diabetes, 5.7 percent is the typical A1C target. Medical professionals recommend that people with diabetes aim for A1C levels of 7 percent or lower, a target associated with fewer diabetes-related complications. However, common approaches to treatment, which typically involve self-administering insulin through multiple daily injections or an insulin pump, do not make that target achievable for many.[11] Despite the known difficulties of reaching the 7 percent target, many people with T1D experience judgment from clinicians for their failure to maintain this standard. Carolyn, a diabetes blogger and manager of a diabetes support group who had been living with T1D for more than fifty years, discussed her frustration with the blame placed on many people with T1D. She suggested that clinicians fail to take into account the cognitive, physical, and emotional toll that constant management can take on a person. She told me:

> And, yes, [people with T1D] are blamed. And even if they're not doing everything they should and could be doing, they're not evil people. They're just burned out. They're tired. They're overwhelmed by it. And how do you keep doing the same thing, and not getting good results, and keep caring to do it?

In this section, I trace how overpromised and underdelivered technological cures and strained clinical relationships contribute to motivations to pursue DIY options for T1D management.

"Everything Is Always Five Years Away": Abandoning the Curative Promise

Despite the weight of blame off-loaded onto people with T1D, the authority to set research and treatment priorities remains firmly in the hands of medical professionals and technologists. My discussions with people with T1D and analysis of DIY communities revealed how this imbalance produces a fundamental tension between professionals and people living with T1D. While many of the informants expressed a desire for better quality of life, clinicians and device manufacturers were preoccupied with a curative promise. In other words, while people with T1D and their families were looking for strategies, practices, and technologies for living better, they instead received promises of an imminent cure. Evelyn, a pharmacist who has lived with T1D for more than thirty years, spoke sardonically about the lifetime of promises that a cure is coming, joking that "everything's always five years away."

Carolyn, however, was adamant about the danger of such a promise. As discussed in the Introduction, she recalled her diagnosis over fifty years ago, which was accompanied by her physician's promise of a forthcoming cure:

> My doctor was world-famous, and he said, "There will be a cure in two years." A lot of us were told that. And after two years, he goes, "No, it'll be five. Don't worry about it." And I started to kind of give up on that after about ten years. I thought, "Well, he's lying."

She went on to say that she fears for people offered the same kind of technological optimism today: "What I hear a lot now in young people is they don't feel they have to control things, because there will be a cure. So, they'll just run wild until then." In Carolyn's estimation, a technological savior is particularly attractive for people managing diabetes, which requires a significant amount of physical and cognitive work:

> Control your portions, and do this and do that, and take shots, and stick things in you, for the benefit of not dying. It's not like, for the benefit of making a million dollars. Or benefit of, you get to eat cookies. You don't. The benefit is, you don't die, and you don't get miserable complications. It's a negative.

The emphasis on cure often prioritizes bench research that rarely materializes into commercial applications. This means that the diabetes technologies available to the average person with T1D have not changed radically since the emergence of insulin pumps and CGMs in the late twentieth century. Benjamin, a software engineer who had been using a pump since he was a preteen, noted that prior to discovering the DIY community, he avoided news about diabetes tech altogether: "I think it's that we were, that it wasn't—I don't want to say hopeless, but it was a fixed set of options. . . . This is what it is to have diabetes." This feeling of stagnation permeated many of the pre-DIY experiences shared by informants. Gordon, father of a young daughter with T1D and employed by a diabetes technology company, suggested that this sense of inaction keeps control and authority firmly in the hands of clinicians and researchers. He asserted that the movement away from a curative promise and toward attentiveness to quality of life enabled participation from people previously excluded from design and care:

> I mean, even just this insight of like, the shift from quality of life to cure, I think is really critical. Because cure is so inaccessible, like it's the specialized guild and priesthood of medicine that has all these boundaries around it that you can't cross.

Quality of life thinking delegates agency back to individuals whose lived experience is essential for meaningful design and practice. When deciding to build and use DIY technologies to manage diabetes, many informants found a dearth of resources, support, and technologies available through sanctioned routes of care. For many, a primary motivator was that the technology they had access to could not provide the features they needed. Further, clinicians failed to provide support or information that could be meaningfully applied to their lives. And yet, in traditional care pathways, despite insufficient technologies and clinical support, informants were still often blamed for their poor outcomes. Their discontent stemmed from perceived invalidation of their experiences and disjunctions between their lived realities and the priorities of clinicians and device manufacturers. These tensions eventually built to such a level that occupying the patient role, in which they were simultaneously responsible and disempowered, was no longer a viable option.

"To Think Less about Staying Alive": Choosing DIY

Evelyn was motivated to pursue DIY options by unsatisfactory interactions with clinicians, especially those who blamed her for her poor quality of life as she worked to manage her diabetes:

> They just didn't have a level of knowledge, I guess is what I would say. I just didn't feel like I was getting anything at all from them. And I was still trying to get something from them. . . . And so, I kept trying to find somebody with the knowledge I needed to make things better, and there was nobody.

When I asked informants about broaching the topic of DIY technology with their clinicians, they shared a range of clinician responses, from disinterest to enthusiasm. Some informants suggested that specialists like endocrinologists often displayed reluctance, while generalists showed interest and even support. Support professionals such as certified diabetes educators, who often had diabetes themselves, were reported to be especially supportive of DIY technologies. Many informants, including Ramona, Erica, Abene, and James, were met with enthusiasm and encouragement from their clinicians, even if they were legally not able to provide much support. Nikol and Jonas in the Czech Republic recalled being asked if they were crazy by a clinician when they requested a loopable pump for their seven-year-old son. They, Marianne (also a parent), and Evelyn all recounted being told that their clinicians could not or would not provide support if they did not follow clinical recommendations. "I can't help you with settings if you keep doing that," an endocrinologist told Marianne, who used DIYAPS with her seven-year-old in Austria.

More often, however, clinicians reacted with disinterest. Melody, an American woman in her mid-thirties, shared her endocrinologist's response when she first showed him a DIY system:

> And I went to the endo's office, and I was like "Hey, I built this thing . . . it's fabulous!" And I was so excited. And he looked at me and said "Okay, do you get less lows?" And I said "Uh, yeah." And he said, "Okay, what prescriptions do you need?" Like, I built this thing, and it's amazing, and you're not interested at all. It's very deflating and disappointing.

Joel, a PhD student with T1D working for a diabetes technology company in California, echoed this frustration. He found DIYAPS after his endocrinologist chastised him about his health without providing alternative approaches. He shared that the endocrinologist "didn't seem very interested in discussing advanced moves in diabetes management. I don't know what he expected me to do."

While less explicitly than in the interviews, the documentation from the DIY community also suggested frustration with the mismatched priorities of commercial manufacturers. For example, DIYAPS relies on communication between a user's CGM and insulin pump, communication made possible through a security gap that commercial manufacturers are actively trying to close. Because of this, some DIYAPS users must rely on older, secondhand pumps. Others must carefully pore over every software update to be sure that their systems will still be usable. One DIY system's documentation addressed the lack of support from commercial manufacturers to allow for communication between devices:

> Until and unless companies elect to provide such access, the open-source community will continue reverse engineering additional insulin pumps wherever possible to make APS technology as widely available as possible until all individuals living with Type 1 Diabetes have the opportunity to sleep safely every night.

Additionally, the recognition and appreciation of a shared lived experience in the design and use of DIYAPS was central to users' decisions to opt for DIY, in direct opposition to the interests of device manufacturers. As Evelyn said:

> My motivation and the motivation of people in the DIY community is parallel. My motivation and the motivation of Dexcom [manufacturer of a popular continuous glucose monitor] are not, because they are a publicly traded company, so automatically our interests are not the same.

Most prominent in those shared motivations was the desire to limit the intense burden of constant disease management, which encompasses both the cognitive weight of decision-making (often involving mathematical calculations and guesswork) and the emotional impact of being solely responsible for the outcomes. "A big reason why people, me included, want to do looping," Gary stated flatly, "is to think less about staying alive." This motivation for adopting DIY technologies should be distinguished from the quality of life dimensions enabled by better management, such as sleep quality. Here, the desirable element of DIY technologies is not that they work better than commercially available management options in terms of clinically relevant measurements such as A1C (although preliminary research suggests this is likely to be the case), but that they reduce the cognitive burden of constant decision-making. As articulated above, this burden is not limited to in-the-moment cognitive processes; it also includes the guilt and blame associated with what clinicians perceive as poor outcomes. By displacing the responsibility of immediate management decisions to the algorithm and shifting focus to oversight of the technology, users distance themselves from those decisions in a way that reduces the emotional impacts of less-than-desirable outcomes. "It takes those decisions that you would make minute by minute, it takes out the emotional payload from that decision, and it does it," Evelyn said, exemplifying this rearticulation of roles and responsibilities in day-to-day management. As Carolyn noted:

> There's really very few, if any, other diseases that are this user-intensive and complicated. And no matter what you do, you're not going to get the same results. So, it's terribly frustrating. . . . When I talked to the researchers, I said, "I want you to understand. This is hard. This isn't like, what pen or pencil am I going to buy?" It's life-and-death decisions that normal people are making. And they're making it every day, and they're choosing to keep involved. It's exhausting.

In addition to making clear the motivation behind many users' decisions to adopt DIY technologies, Carolyn's statement exposes another disjunction: People who are not engaged in the day-to-day work of T1D do not have the same framework for understanding diabetes management choices as those who are. Gordon recalled:

> What we found to my great frustration and anger was that when we tried to talk about the actual burden of care, people denied it. People who had no engagement with us said that can't be. . . . It was very, very upsetting. Basically, within the first month we just learned to stop talking about it in public because we didn't have the emotional capacity to not lose it on these people who were denying our experience from nothing.

Because DIYAPS is rooted in those embodied experiences, it offers not only practical solutions that resonate with the expressed needs of people with T1D but also affective support and validation, as discussed further below.

For many informants, the displacing of the everyday decision-making of diabetes management to the DIY algorithm was equally as important as—if not more important than—perceptible differences in the clinical measurements of diabetes, such as A1C levels. Aditi, a physician and mother of a young son using a DIY system in the United Kingdom, found that she was more concerned with the "burden of [management]" and the "constant decision-making" than with any specific clinical outcome. She told me:

> I would take away the burden rather than the blood glucose levels. Yes, it's nice to be in range. Yes, it's nice to be in range more and more, but my worry about diabetes management in the long run is the burden of diabetes management, not the actual levels of glucose.

"The word 'control' is so significant in the diabetes world," Carolyn observed, and nearly all of the interviews featured themes around control: over diabetes, over management plans, over biometric data. Many informants directly connected control to quality of life and quality of life to the adoption of DIY technologies. As noted above, the distinction between tools and technologies that support quality of life and those deployed for curative purposes is felt acutely by many with T1D, with the latter being positioned as an elusive but alluring promise in the medical establishment. For some informants, control over their management plans translated into freedom. As Abene, a PhD student in Spain, put it, upon beginning to use DIY remote monitoring of her blood sugar levels, "I felt more independent than I used to be." For Czech parents Nikol and Jonas, whose seven-year-old son had been living with T1D for five years, "the remote control, it is again a big step because when our son wants to go with his friends, for example, we have him under control, so we don't have to be on the phone with the parents of the friends every five minutes."

An additional vector of control enabled by DIYAPS comes in the form of biometric data, in response to the proprietary hoarding of information that characterizes commercial products. DIY, in contrast, is committed to transparency. Gordon emphasized this foundational value, sharing that because members of this community have experienced technological blackboxing, loss of access to their health data, and relegation to submissive patient roles, the technology and the community have been developed to intentionally push back against those experiences and reclaim agency.[12] When speaking about a company formalizing DIY technology for regulatory approval, he noted the values it strove to maintain:

> Of being radically open and transparent, that people own their own data and should be able to both understand how it's being used and controlled. And those are not common values in technology. I think that comes from this lived experience and intentionally shaping the company to exist to serve these values and these goals, as opposed to get acquired or ship a product real fast.

The visibility of data enabled by DIYAPS creates a perception of control by virtue of the transparency of the decisions the algorithm makes. This takes diabetes management out of the black box of commercial devices and out of the guesswork of analog interventions such as multiple daily injections. As Benjamin said, "I think about my blood sugar more, and yet I think about it less."

Erica, a nursing student who had lived with diabetes for more than two decades, recalled of her time prior to using DIYAPS:

> There was a little bit of a cloud over my potential and then all of a sudden it was like the clouds broke apart and moved and I really feel like I'm fully living my life. My brain and my body and my energy. Everything's very clear, very definitive now. Like there's nothing that I feel like I can't do because I actually am in it.

Ultimately, and in direct contradiction to clinical expectations, most informants were not preoccupied with whether DIYAPS enabled better quantitative outcomes; rather, they were interested in whether it helped them live better.

Reimagining Risk and Responsibility in DIY Diabetes Tech

In 2019, the U.S. Food and Drug Administration published a safety communication for people with T1D and their health care providers, warning against the "use of devices for diabetes management unauthorized for sale in the United States, whether used alone or along with other devices."[13] This statement was issued following a reported incident of an insulin overdose by a DIY user. The user, who required medical intervention, received too much insulin because of some unknown incompatibility between the user's CGM and an "unauthorized" automated insulin dosing algorithm.

While the statement acknowledges that customizability drives people with T1D to pursue "multiple treatment and management options," it cautions that combining devices that have not been tested for compatibility or introducing unauthorized elements like the DIYAPS algorithm produces "new risks . . . that the FDA has not evaluated for safety or effectiveness." The exact nature of the incident is not clear from the statement, and it does not provide information on the rates of severe adverse reactions with authorized diabetes management technologies. Instead, it implies that the "unauthorized" nature of DIY technology is what positions it as inherently risky. In this section, I discuss how the meanings of risk, responsibility, and safety have become fluid and contextual in DIY communities.

"The Disease Is Going to Kill Me If I Don't Do Something": Risks Old and New

Many informants told me that clinicians, manufacturers, regulators, and family members discourage people managing T1D from pursuing DIY options, citing fears for their health and safety. These moments brought into focus how different lived experiences produce different conceptions of risk. I asked each informant if building and using DIY technology ever felt risky, and most reported that people in their lives who were not engaging with diabetes in a sustained way had more concerns about DIY technologies than they did, in part because of a general lack of awareness of the risks in daily management. Abene recounted, "So that's why . . . [my doctor]'s afraid. We're relying on old pumps, so it could happen that they are broken, that the rig will not be working okay. Who knows? It could happen. Of course, it might also happen with my actual pump." By "my actual pump," she meant the pump allocated to her through the Spanish government, and the "old pump" she referred to was the DIYAPS-compatible pump she had purchased online to start looping. While Abene's statement may at first appear blasé, it resonates with the inherent uncertainty in daily diabetes management felt by many informants. Carolyn shared a very similar conversation with her husband when she first started looping: "I didn't have any anxiety or any fear. My husband did. 'How do you know this isn't going to kill you?' And I think my answer might have been, 'Well, the disease is going to kill me if I don't do something.'"

The burden of decision-making in the daily management of diabetes and feelings of guilt and shame at failing to manage appropriately figured heavily in informants' decisions to adopt DIY technology. By displacing immediate decision-making to the system, many people felt emotional and cognitive relief. While those who do not engage in the thousands of daily management decisions related to diabetes perceive the relinquishing of control to an algorithm as potentially risky, many informants expressed the exact opposite. While the guidance documents created by DIY users urge caution and skepticism of the algorithm's decision-making ability, emphasizing that the algorithm cannot learn and relies on accurate input and attention from the user, trust in the algorithm over one's own imperfect decision-making was a strong theme among informants. Melody said, "This is actually safer than me making the decisions when I'm sleep deprived or when I'm not paying attention." Erica had similar feelings, saying that the algorithm "is proving itself to be a better decision-maker than I am." How risk becomes understood is deeply contextual, and the lived experience of diabetes management (and mismanagement) when one is tired, sick, or otherwise distracted shifts that risk calculus toward trusting the DIY technology to take on some of the everyday decision-making.

Risk, especially the differential and contextual risk that accompanies living with a chronic disease, appeared in the documentation as well. "The ultimate answer to 'is it safe,'" one set of DIY guidance documents read, "will be something each individual decides for themselves." This approach to risk differs significantly from that of traditional health care regulation, in which safety and risk are adjudicated exclusively by governance bodies as opposed to individuals (including clinicians and manufacturers). While documents from both within and outside the DIY community recognized the potential risks of DIYAPS, only the informal documents asserted the individual agency of the user to determine whether the benefits are worth the risks. Here also, the difference between "patient" and "individual" should be noted. The formal documents, like the FDA warning quoted above, encouraged the "patient" to take a passive role and rely on clinical and regulatory guidance, while the DIY documentation noted the right of the "individual" to decide what risks are allowable. The latter also diverged from the homogeneous and universal "patient" of regulatory documentation in recognizing the importance of individual experience, meaning there is no one right answer for the community at large. With this individualization of risk emerged a sense of individual responsibility as well.

Many informants touched on the individual responsibilities that arise from pursuing DIY technologies, which were distinct from the more general responsibilities of diabetes management. Much of this new dimension of responsibility comes from the lack of a formal support network within DIY spaces. As Melody stated, "If you do use it, know that if it breaks, you'll have to fix it. You can ask for help, but sometimes people are living their lives." The analyzed guidance documents echoed these sentiments, with statements such as "You really need to figure this out yourself" commonly appearing. Parents Nikol and Jonas expressed this perception of personal responsibility as tangibly different from their experience of commercial products, where a customer service representative or clinician could provide guidance and direction at any time. Nikol noted that with DIY, "everyone has a different experience, and no one is a responsible person." Jonas added, "Only we are responsible because we have decided to use the application."

Informants' acknowledgments of responsibility were always accompanied by emphatic assertions of the benefits they gained by taking that responsibility. In other words, they overwhelmingly agreed that the results were worth the risks.

"We Care about Safety": Ambivalence toward Regulation

Informants often held multiple, sometimes conflicting, perspectives on the design and regulation of medical devices such as insulin pumps and CGMs. While several expressed frustration at the slow and rigid approval processes that prevent medical devices and systems like DIYAPS from being commercially available, the majority also said that they trusted regulatory bodies and their safety approval processes. Both Benjamin and Nikol, for example, stated an interest in adopting commercial hybrid closed-loop devices once they become available and approved by regulatory bodies, in part because this would mitigate the responsibility that DIY solutions demand. Joel struggled to strike a balance between safety and customizability, noting:

> I guess that is my fear, because I do feel like obviously you can iterate a lot faster and make more individualized solutions when you have more control like with the DIY stuff. I expect a lot of that to go away, and that is a trade-off because supposedly the solutions coming out will be broadly safer, but they won't be as customizable, I assume.

Other informants' fears regarding regulation were more immediate. Amy, mother of a preteen with T1D and employee of a diabetes technology company, mentioned she was initially afraid to adopt a DIY system for her daughter because she did not want to be accused of negligence for using an off-label treatment. Carolyn revealed that she no longer shared public information online about looping because she worried that her Medicare benefits might be affected. Evelyn feared the regulatory community could partner with device manufacturers to further limit access to the materials necessary to DIY. Her anxieties about regulatory gatekeeping were bolstered by the 2019 U.S. recall of Medtronic MiniMed 508 and Paradigm series insulin pumps because of a security flaw in the pumps' wireless communications—the flaw that enabled them to be used in DIY systems.[14] However, informants did not interpret all communications from regulators regarding DIY systems as threatening. Melody shared her thoughts on the 2019 FDA statement warning about the use of DIY systems and devices, noting that she viewed it not as a threat to DIY communities but as an affirmation of the regulators' commitment to safety:

> We care about safety, and so we absolutely support people reporting to the community or FDA if they have problems. (Interestingly, a lot of people learned through this communication that you can/should report commercial adverse events, too—many people don't know that! So adverse events go underreported even for commercial devices.)[15]

DIYers have at times been presented in the media as radically opposed to the "common sense" of regulatory and authority bodies. The statements quoted above, however, along with the fact that some informants were hoping for (or working toward) regulatory approval for DIY systems, resist this narrative, configuring

DIY communities as responsible users invested in regulatory approval as a means to expand the reach of DIY solutions.

Additionally, calls for regulation and formalization of resources appeared throughout the interviews. Users were especially interested in commercialization as an opportunity to gain formal networks of support, akin to customer service, for emerging management solutions like DIYAPS. As Gary shared, users' need for more support applied not only to DIY systems but also more broadly to other complex medical devices coming to market:

> And I think as these systems become more and more complex, the FDA needs to look at whether it is realistic for someone of average intelligence and self-awareness—whether the amount of training materials provided is sufficient, only relying on those materials. I think it is too much to ask a patient to have to rely on unofficial sources to get the most out of these systems.

Here, regulation was not seen as an impediment to innovation but as an essential component of making these innovations accessible to a diverse set of users.

Regulation was also a major theme in the documentation. As with the interviews, some of the materials described it as a necessary safeguard. For example, one document asserted, "It is critically important that you only use a tested, fully functioning FDA or CE approved insulin pump and CGM for closing an automated insulin dosing loop."[16] Others viewed regulation as an impediment to access. One blog accompanying a DIY system's documentation addressed this in justifying DIY: "We believe that we can make safe and effective APS technology available more quickly, to more people, rather than just waiting for current APS efforts to complete clinical trials and be FDA-approved and commercialized through traditional processes." This ambivalent and precarious relationship with manufacturers and regulators, acknowledging both their value and their shortcomings, characterized the attitudes of many in the DIY community.

Embodied Resistance through Community

"Rogue cowboy hackers . . . ," Evelyn laughed, "that's what Dexcom called us, back in the beginning." While Dexcom, the manufacturer of a commonly used continuous glucose monitor, apparently leveraged the term "hacker" derogatorily, informants explicitly or implicitly all advocated for principles often related to the "hacker ethic," including collaboration, experimentation, altruism, and radical transparency.[17] Others found the allure of building and creating new technologies exciting. "It got my 'gadget-drive' going," Benjamin said. "It felt like a new toy, in a lot of ways, but so much more." For Ramona, a medical student living in southeastern Europe, the process was "like an adventure." The twin desires for community and agency that articulate the DIY experience diverge significantly from the isolated, obedient patient role that disabled and chronically ill people are expected to assume in Western medicine. This hacker ethos draws many to DIY spaces, which offer a contrast to the often-invalidating encounters of the clinic.

In this section, I focus on the emergence of a cohesive community within the DIYAPS movement. Key to this process is the reclamation of agency among DIY users who reject a submissive patient role in favor of becoming agential actors. Additionally, foundational to the community ethos that undergirds the open-access nature of DIYAPS is the privileging and validation of lived experience, particularly in response to the epistemic invalidation that permeates clinical interactions. Third, the articulation of a supportive DIY community transformed many informants' perceptions of their disabled and/or chronically ill identities. Finally, despite a strong community ethos, a number of fissures exist both within the DIY community and between the DIY community and the larger population of people with T1D, in part exacerbated by assumptions about engagement, knowledge, and motivation. Ultimately, the solidification of a coherent DIY community counteracts the hyperindividualization and pathologization of diabetes that characterize Western medicine, opening up generative new understandings of what it means to live with chronic illness.

From Passive Patient to "Rogue Cowboy Hacker"

The iterative, organic, and experimental elements of DIYAPS featured in many interviews. James, a retiree in the United Kingdom who had lived with T1D for more than forty years, found the playfulness of DIY appealing. He stated that whenever he had a question about what DIYAPS could do and he could not find a readily available answer, he thought, "'Okay, nobody knows about this.'

And, you know, I'm techie, I play. I go, 'What happens if I do this? Or what happens if I do that?'" Melody also alluded to an openness to exploration as necessary to making DIY work:

> So, it wasn't so much that I knew a solution, like "Oh, we're going to do X and Y and Z" and you know, be really straightforward and easy. It was experimentation . . . and just chipping away until we figured out how to do it.

The experimental and self-reliant nature of the DIY community also leads users to become invested in both the technology and the individual successes of others in the community. As Gordon said:

> I call it out as the Ikea effect: where you spend time making that awful shelf. Even if it's falling apart and has real problems, you love it because you put time and blood, sweat, and tears into it. It's something I think about a great deal as we watch the community online grow.

This collective buy-in promotes a culture that is committed to iterative improvements, knowledge and resource sharing, and mutual encouragement. Such encouragement extends to user networks for sharing supplies and resources. Erica, for example, told me that she receives many of her necessary supplies from friends in the DIY and broader T1D community, as they are not covered by her insurance: "Everyone is with you to have the best management possible." In 2023, close to half of people with diabetes in a U.S.-based study reported running out of necessary supplies such as CGM sensors or lancets, and more than three-quarters reported issues with access to insulin and its affordability. More than a third said that they relied on "compensatory strategies" such as rationing insulin, trading supplies, or seeking donations.[18] Under these conditions, community can be necessary for survival.

Inherent in conversations about experimentation with DIYAPS were acknowledgments of collaboration, both within the DIY community itself and with other stakeholders, such as commercial device manufacturers and researchers. Informants viewed openness, transparency, and knowledge sharing as vital for the development of the DIY community as well as for increasing DIY accessibility to others through regulatory approval and commercialization.

"I believe the technology people actually are trying to develop something that helps diabetics," Carolyn shared when explaining why she engages with commercial device manufacturers. "So I want to give them access. I want them to be able to talk to me. I want to be able to give them input. And I just, somehow, plow forward." In her estimation, commercial manufacturers are well-intentioned but uninformed, and so she makes a concerted effort to develop collaborations, injecting herself into the process often without invitation. Melody also articulated the importance of collaboration across stakeholders, advocating for radical transparency and the centering of the experiences of users with T1D as crucial to meaningful technological development:

> We don't necessarily have to work with companies, though we'd like to. We don't have to work with researchers, though we'd like to, but it's like how do we get everybody all together? So social media and kind of the open-source diabetes community has played an interesting role in all these areas, including research of how to bring people together instead of talking over each other's heads or duplicating work or you know focusing on credentials or whatever. We can actually say, "What are the unsolved problems that are actually meaningful to the community and let's go tackle those." Because that's good for the diabetes community, it's great for the researchers and their careers, it's great for medical literature in the long term. So how do we combine all these things to be a win-win-win all around.

The hacker ethic that infused interviews was also present in much of the documentation, primarily through references to collaboration, transparency, and iteration. "Using [DIYAPS] is essentially carrying out a medical experiment on yourself," one guidance document stated, while another asserted, "Individuals . . . are essentially doing an (n = 1) experiment, which they have a right to do by themselves." Transparency in how an algorithm works, who contributed to creating it (one site featured a long list of names that ran several pages), and other details establishes a sense of trustworthiness: There can be no blackboxing the technological processes because users need to build their systems themselves.

"[DIYAPS] is open and transparent in how it works," one document read, qualifying that transparency to move beyond traditional expertise by noting that DIYAPS is designed to be "understandable not just by experts, but also by clinicians and end users (patients)." The documentation recognized people with T1D first and foremost as users of this technology, rather than immediately slotting them into a submissive patient role. Further, many of the documents highlighted and encouraged collaborative efforts—between open-source projects and among traditional researchers, manufacturers, and users. The documentation for all three DIY systems included examples of how users might contribute to the broader DIY community. Options ranged from contributing to software development to providing language translations to donating money, supplies, or data. All of these documents emphasized that everyone has a place and something to contribute.

This hacker ethic is in direct conflict with the clinical responses to DIY experienced by many DIY users. When people with T1D and their families are held responsible for poor health outcomes but receive little to no support, and sometimes outright resistance, for pursuing new types of off-label management plans like DIYAPS, they find themselves caught in a bind in which they are configured as both accountable and impotent in clinical settings. The DIY community provides an alternative set of power dynamics that still configures them as responsible but also enables them to make meaningful decisions about how they manage their diabetes.

"I Know My Body": Valuing Shared Experiential Knowledge

Both informants and guidance documents highlighted the ways in which embodied and experiential knowledge is leveraged in DIY communities to resist and transform the invalidating and insufficient paradigms in traditional medical interactions. As discussed in previous sections, informants expressed trust in and affinity for DIY communities in part because of their shared experiences and motivations, and in part because of the allure and excitement of creating, collaborating on, and experimenting with off-label treatments. Additionally, informants described the value of these DIY technologies in terms of quality of life and reduction of cognitive burden, two elements of living with diabetes that are often unacknowledged or undervalued in traditional clinical interactions. In direct opposition to perceptions of distrust and mismatched priorities with commercial device manufacturers and clinicians, the majority of informants explicitly stated that their trust in DIY communities emerged from their common experiences and priorities. Amy stated, "I think that the shared experiences bring us together and we have to be compassionate for one another, because we're not always compassionate to ourselves."

Members of DIY communities live with diabetes on a daily basis, and this became a source of trust for many informants. This aligned with their distrust or dismissal of clinical and manufacturer knowledge as being incomplete. Gary shared:

> And a lot of health care providers don't have diabetes themselves, so they don't understand what it's like living with it. . . . Because all physicians can learn through word of mouth and studies, but if you're not living—diabetes is about the most intensive, hands-on disease there is. You have to do so much self-care.

He continued by asserting that people must rely on informal communities of people with diabetes in part because traditional medical training makes it very difficult for people with T1D to become clinicians. The DIY community, however, celebrates the expertise of everyday practice. Built on a foundation of flexibility and individual customizability, DIYAPS communities adhere to the basic principle that, as Benjamin put it, "I know my body. And I know what works for me."

It is important to note here the distinction between the embodied knowledge of people with T1D and the experiential knowledge of guardians of children with T1D, a division acutely felt by several guardians who were interviewed. "There's even a sheer between my experience as a parent caring for a child and the experience of somebody who actually lives with the disease," Gordon noted when discussing his involvement with a design project centering the experiences of a teen with T1D. He continued:

> And I think it's an important distinction to hold. I consider myself a part of the type 1 community, but I do not carry the disease in my body. I carry the burden of that disease for my daughter but one day she's going to take it and be the primary one carrying it. It's a bit of an insider–outsider perspective.

Marianne and Amy both also addressed their role as parents of children with diabetes as one distinct from that of people managing their own diabetes. Marianne shared that while her young son was currently using DIY technologies and starting to become involved in his own management, he had the right to choose what he wanted to do in the future. Amy acknowledged her daughter's frustration at times, admitting, "As much as I want to be there for my daughter, I'm not the one going through it." This distinction highlights the informants' recognition and respect for the embodied knowledge of people with T1D as well as the practical and experiential knowledge of guardians and caretakers of children with T1D. While parents overwhelmingly expressed feeling an immense responsibility for their children's management, they emphasized that they themselves do not physically experience, in Erica's words, "the extreme rollercoaster that diabetes can be sometimes." It is unclear from this research whether fissures have formed between guardians of children with T1D and adults with T1D, although other research addressing disability advocacy more broadly suggests that significant tensions sometimes arise between parent-led and advocate-led social movements, particularly when priorities and experiences diverge.[19]

The privileging and centering of embodied and experiential knowledge also served to transform informants' personal relationships with diabetes. Many recalled growing up feeling isolated or stigmatized because of their diabetes, which in turn caused them to distance themselves from it and its management at some point in their lives. Benjamin said that he avoided forums for communicating with other people with T1D because "I didn't want to define myself by diabetes." Joel had taken a similar position before he found the DIY diabetes community: "I think I was always more or less trying to minimize the amount of time that I . . . I didn't really identify having diabetes as part of my identity."

Parents of young children with diabetes observed this process of alienation. Nikol, whose seven-year-old son had just started using DIYAPS earlier that year, noted that he was currently experiencing the realization of difference that many of the adults with T1D recounted in their interviews. "So, I think for him it was a very big moment," Nikol said, "when he was thinking that 'I am a bit different than the others.' I don't think he was thinking any of that before."

For many informants, their introduction into DIY communities altered their relationship to diabetes as well as their relationships to others. Melody articulated this transition:

> I do consider diabetes to be a chronic disease, and that is something that, like, yes, I would say I have a chronic disease. It has always been a part of my identity, that's actually something I was very concerned about when I was diagnosed. I didn't want it to be part of my identity, I didn't want to be thought of as a person with diabetes, um, but I just feel so differently now. I don't want to be cliched like "I feel so empowered now"—it's not like I wasn't empowered before, but I just feel more confident, is probably the right word, in terms of living life with diabetes and figuring things out and going with the flow and having the tools to support me to do all those things.

Several informants expressed similar feelings of empowerment or confidence, evolving from a sense of impotence or powerlessness in clinical engagements. Carolyn shared: "That's part of the blessing of the do-it-yourself community, is it's impatient. And it's not . . . I don't know if I'd say it's angry, but it's just impatient. It's like, 'Okay, don't tell us to wait.' So, I like that." This statement, most likely in reference to the hashtag #WeAreNotWaiting, which is often used as a mantra within the DIYAPS community, suggests the empowerment, collective motivation, and action-oriented ethos that make DIYAPS appealing. For many, involvement in a like-minded community was as valuable as the technology itself. Gordon was even more explicit about the transformation of his perception of himself in relation to his young daughter's diabetes:

> I can tell you, like [DIYAPS] and finding that group of people that's transformative for my own sense of agency and well-being and of not just giving up and moving beyond victimhood and back into agency. And even if it's not effective for anything else, that's really valuable.

Some informants pointed to how access to both people and resources that redefined diabetes, control, and community reconfigured their attitudes toward themselves and others. Melody, Amy, and Gordon also discussed feeling compelled to bring this community ethos to other disability communities, suggesting an affinity for a broader disabled community rather than a view of people with T1D as singular and exceptional. Melody thought that the support and attention given to the DIYAPS community could be leveraged "into a broader conversation around the broader principles of patient-driven innovation and research." Gordon was slightly more reserved in his opinion on whether the possibilities of DIYAPS could be generalized to other disability communities, but, he said, "I've wanted to try, because I think that there has been so much good about it." The identification with and affinity for broader disability communities signals a movement away from adherence to medical categorization and toward a political and social disability identity, a move that further resists medicalization and clinical authority.

"They Are Afraid to Ask for More": Stratification in the DIY Community

Despite the community ethos that permeated many of the analyzed guidance documents and informants' perceptions of DIY spaces, several fault lines exist both within the DIY community and between DIY users and the population with T1D more broadly. Notably, several informants acknowledged their positions of privilege that allowed them to seek out, build, and maintain DIY systems. The characteristics they mentioned included financial stability, education, community connections, and having the confidence to challenge clinicians. "We're privileged in that we had full-time jobs; we were able to spend our nights and weekends on this as a passion project," Melody immediately noted when asked about the financial and emotional costs of pursing DIY. "Not everybody in these kinds of communities can do that," she told me. "So, we started from a position of privilege in being able to dedicate our time to do that." For some, like Ramona, Carolyn, Benjamin, and Evelyn, being early adopters of diabetes technology predisposed them to be curious about DIYAPS. "I've always been a little ahead of the game," Benjamin joked, sharing that he had first started using an insulin pump in the 1990s as a child, much to the surprise of his endocrinologist. Others had backgrounds in technology that made them feel comfortable building and using DIY systems.

Interestingly, being perceived by clinicians as particularly adept with technology predisposed many informants to move away from commercial products to DIY systems. "You're the kind of patient we like to have," Benjamin recalled being told by an endocrinologist, guessing it was "because I'm knowledgeable about care and I'm active in the process. As opposed to saying, 'Hey, this is what's wrong with me, what do I do?'" Ironically, being identified as "good patients" pushed many informants into more agential, less clinically compliant roles.

Nikol and Jonas, who were initially discouraged and scolded by their clinician for requesting an insulin pump for their young son whose diabetes was not well controlled, were eventually told by another clinician, "I will give it to you because I can see that you are smart enough to operate it and to have it under control." Ramona shared that her clinician approved of her curiosity around other management options: "She was very excited and happy and she's like, 'Oh my God, you are the ideal patient.'" Being "advanced," "active," or "engaged" with care was a common theme among informants, creating a sense that they recognized themselves as different from others managing diabetes, which imparted a confidence to explore DIY options and challenge clinicians.

The appearance of the "advanced user" narrative raises questions about the position of people not deemed advanced users by the medical establishment. As Gordon noted:

> There is this myth among clinicians that pumps and CGMs are for advanced users, that you really should prove that you can do it the hard way first before we can trust you with a pump. And that's like saying, you got to learn how to drive a stick shift before I let you drive a car. We might have a better time if we gave people easier-to-drive cars that they need to live.

Despite this rejection of the arbitrary distinction between average and advanced users, all informants spoke not just about their own experiences with DIY but also about their perceptions concerning who should or can DIY responsibly. When I asked James, for example, if there were people who could benefit from DIYAPS who felt intimidated or unable to access it because of the technical or knowledge requirements, he answered bluntly, "I think there are, yes. But hey, which way do you go? Stupid dead people or alive people who may not have as good control?" Such responses, which in some ways ran counter to the affirmation that the benefits of DIY should be available to all people, were often inflected with assumptions about the motivations, engagement levels, and attention to detail deemed necessary for success with DIY. Nikol suggested that there are many people who could benefit from DIY, but their passivity and unwillingness to seek out alternative approaches prevent them from achieving what she and her family have achieved. "But there are people who are in the same situation we were five years ago," she said:

> And they don't have enough energy, or they are not such [people], so they are afraid to go somewhere and ask someone for help or something. They are just living with what the city is giving to them. What the place and the situation is giving to them. And they are afraid to ask for more. So, our advantage is we are not so afraid.

Gordon also noted a passivity in mainstream diabetes communities, which typically mobilized around fundraising for medical research rather than around action-oriented solutions such as DIY. "Yeah, it feels like church," he joked, referring to fundraising events common in diabetes communities:

> I mean, I grew up in church and I still go to church. And it feels like this is what we're supposed to do. Like the families with type 1, you go to type 1 runs and you build a team, and you raise the money. This is what we all do together. And that's not bad . . . [but] I found patterns of passivity and acceptance and consolation and community.

Gary, who did not receive a T1D diagnosis until adulthood, also suggested that many people are passive about their treatment plans or content with suboptimal outcomes, particularly those who have been managing their diabetes for a long time. "The strange paradox," he observed, "is that often people who have had diabetes for a very long time, they fall into very old habits that are not optimal." Many informants mentioned that DIY systems are, in Carolyn's words, "not the appropriate forum" for everyone, and their judgments of passivity and lack of self-motivation were often tempered with understanding about the difficulties of day-to-day diabetes management. Recognizing that not all people managing T1D have the bandwidth, time, or energy to pursue DIY technologies, they did not harshly dismiss those who chose other paths. As Melody noted, "For the most part it's not a knowledge gap so much as an experience gap and . . . people will choose to close [the loop] at different times."

That a lack of technical competence is a potential barrier to entry was adamantly refuted by both informants and the documentation. Erica, when recalling her first impressions of DIYAPS, stated:

> I was super intimidated by it. I was so intimidated 'cause I was like, "Yeah, I've just been HTML coding for like, a hot second in my life, but what does it mean . . ." The way that I think about do-it-yourself technology is I, fully in my brain, the only way I make it make sense is to say that you're "hacking" into the medical devices. And that's such a scary thing to say, even now, and I'm wearing them all over me.

Her initial feeling that DIY required technical competence beyond her ability was common among informants, who also said they eventually realized this was not the case. Nearly all asserted that the technical skills needed to pursue DIY systems are not actually a significant barrier, despite their previous assumptions. Later in our conversation, Erica said, "I think the biggest—one of the biggest misnomers of do-it-yourself is that you have to have any knowledge of coding. Because what you need to be able to do is copy and paste. And everyone, except for maybe my dad, can do that." Others concurred. Melody recalled discussion among community members:

> We also started having lots of conversations around access. I wasn't comfortable with—and other people weren't either—that only technical people could figure out how to do it. And so, we started writing some documentation. And we constantly over the last three and a half years have really had a conversation around [it]—and it's evolved.

James found the conversational and welcoming nature of the documentation appealing, saying that it was "obviously written from somebody who was type 1, rather than somebody who was a techie."

While much of the documentation was written in an informal

tone that cultivated a sense of community, in several instances "developers" were distinguished from "users," indicating a hierarchical structure. One set of documentation referred continually to "you" (the end user) and "we" (the developers), despite an invitation to users to edit the materials. Another document requested donations to go "towards the developers' costs to leave their darkened rooms and meet each other at conferences and events to let their creative and analytical brains bounce off each other." These distinctions in the documentation hint at tacit separation within the community.

Although generally informants agreed that technical ability was not a serious barrier to entry, there was still an implicit expectation in the community that members enter with a basic understanding of the technologies and access to technological resources. Aditi, for example, found members of the community to be quite resistant to providing assistance to those perceived as "non-techie." She said:

> I can see the frustration where a lot of the techie people are just saying, "Read the docs, read the docs, read the docs," as answers to questions. And some of the questions, okay, could have been answered from the first few lines of the documents. But actually, the documents are not well written for non-techie people.

Further, assumptions about technical skills may inadvertently alienate people who do not have regular access to the Internet or desktop computers. Additionally, no informants broached the topic of access for people with comorbid disabilities such as vision impairments or issues with fine motor skills. Such consideration is imperative, given the prevalence of these secondary conditions in people with T1D.[20] That these issues were not raised in this set of interviews is not to say that they are of no concern to the DIY community, but it is important to note that a lack of attention to these impacts could reinforce the boundaries of DIY to exclude certain geographies, socioeconomic statuses, and bodyminds that disallow regular computer use.

While most informants dismissed technical knowledge as a barrier, many viewed a different knowledge threshold as necessary for success with DIY: knowledge about diabetes. When asked about technical competence, Melody simply stated, "The more important knowledge is your diabetes." Several informants, including Erica,

James, and Gordon, worried that people who adopted DIYAPS too quickly following diagnosis had not yet learned certain critical skills for diabetes management. These skills enable users to set up their DIY systems appropriately and to treat their diabetes should their systems fail. "I've seen that in diabetics who go on technologies super early," Erica said, comparing their inexperience to her own confidence in managing her diabetes through low-tech treatments like multiple daily injections:

> Like they have a CGM failure, or their insulin pump will break, and they're lost. They don't know how to do a conversion back to like long and fast insulin, right? They don't know how to do those things mathematically or even conceptually. They can't wrap their mind around it, and that to me, is terrifying.

She continued by hypothesizing that one reason some people who try DIY technologies do poorly is that they do not have the requisite knowledge to get their settings correct. Gary, Erica, Melody, James, and Aditi all suggested that fundamental diabetes education, on topics such as carb counting and glucose absorption, is significantly lacking for many people, and this presents a substantial impediment to DIYing as well as to management by traditional means. As Ramona noted, to engage with DIY systems, "you need to have time to study, to understand . . . the information in the system, how it works." So even while "the diversity has absolutely expanded," according to Melody, and DIY users have worked to fill diabetes education gaps, lack of access to knowledge and time remains a significant barrier to entry. While commercialization of DIY systems may in some ways mitigate this barrier, insufficient support and resources on the individual user level means the continuation of disparities between those who can use these systems effectively and those who cannot.

Like many of the informants, the documentation consistently emphasized the work that users must put into DIY. For example, one educational article flatly stated, "'Looping' doesn't stand for 'not doing anything.'" Another set of guidance documents elaborated on this idea: "Implementation requires diligent and consistent testing and monitoring to ensure each piece of the system is monitoring, predicting, and controlling as desired. The performance and quality of your system lies solely with you." Self-motivation, knowledge of diabetes, and work ethic were stressed throughout, constructing the DIY user as curious, hardworking, and self-responsible. Knowledge about diabetes management (including the math that is at the core of the DIYAPS algorithms) was underlined as essential. As with the informants, however, technical competence was not. One set of guidance documents offered reassurance: "It is totally understandable to be intimidated and worried that this will be too technical . . . but please realize that this is actually as simple as reading, copying a few lines and clicking a few buttons . . . REALLY." Like the informants, the documentation writers seemed to be aware that presumptions about technical prowess might discourage some potential DIY users, so they threaded welcoming and supportive statements throughout. Such statements may serve to counteract the advanced user myth, while emphasis on self-motivation and responsibility may feed it.

Reclaiming Agency with Do-It-Yourself Artificial Pancreas Systems

In this chapter, I have explored the perceived authoritative and bodily transgressions committed by DIY diabetes tech communities in an effort to demand a recognition of lived expertise in the face of systemic clinical invalidation. These transgressions fall into three broad categories: eschewing a curative promise in favor of addressing quality of life, reimagining risk in a bodymind made inherently risky by disabled embodiment, and rejecting the hyper-individualization of medicalization in favor of community ethos. Taken together, they mark a rejection of the submissive patient role prescribed to disabled and chronically ill people and represent a threat to the authority over disabled embodiment claimed by clinicians and technologists. In this section, I examine these transgressions more closely before turning to the ways in which race, gender, and class inflect the construction of DIY communities.

Transgressive Hopes

The promise of a cure for type 1 diabetes hangs over most clinical interactions. By positioning a cure as imminent but mediated through clinical and commercial outlets, medical professionals and technologists retain their authority over diabetes. Curative logics, driven by an assumption that able-bodiedness is both preferred and morally superior, undergird modern Western medicine. Privileging highly individualistic and medical interventions for disability produces conditions under which "disability" is understood to mean nonnormative or maladaptive biological structures. Disability becomes discrete, identifiable, and treatable through scientific and medical regimens, and so nonbiological experiences, such as the cognitive burden of daily management, become buried beneath the pursuit for able-bodiedness. However, as Gordon noted, the shift away from curative promises and toward the many meanings and nuances of quality of life signaled an abandonment of deference to professional expertise. Understanding quality of life demands a deep and sustained engagement with lived experience—an acknowledgment of embodied expertise and disabled knowledge.

The distinction between DIYAPS and commercially available diabetes management technologies may be best articulated through what Aimi Hamraie and Kelly Fritsch describe as the distinction between "disability technoscience" and "crip technoscience." They operate under the base assumption that "disabled people are experts and designers of everyday life," rather than passive subjects that have material and social reality enacted on them.[21] They adhere to an understanding of disability as a site of cultural and knowledge formations:

> Unlike typical approaches to disability that objectify disabled people and situate expertise in medical professionals and nondisabled designers or engineers, crip technoscience posits that disabled people are active participants in the design of everyday life. Not only do disabled people make access in our everyday lives in ways that do not get recognized as design, but the lived experience of disability, and the shared experience of disability community creates specific expertise and knowledge that informs technoscientific practices.[22]

The unique knowledge that disabled people can leverage has been operationalized in various forms of technological intervention, often through off-label, hacked, or other uses not endorsed by medical and political authorities. This is in direct response and opposition to "disability technoscience," which is deployed against disabled bodyminds as a means to cure, intervene, or otherwise condemn. Crip technoscience rejects this construction in favor of disabled knowledge production. DIYAPS is reminiscent of what M. Remi Yergeau describes as "criptastic hacking," a process by which disabled people "are the movers, not the moved-upon. We are the ones who should be hacking spaces and oppressive social systems; we should *not* have our bodies and our brains hacked upon by non-disabled people."[23] Invoking Yergeau, Hamraie and Fritsch write that "criptastic hacking highlights crip technoscience as a field of relations, knowledges, and practices that enables the flourishing of crip ways of producing and engaging the material world."[24] This resonates strongly with Gordon's assertion that the limited engagement of people with diabetes in the design process for diabetes technologies has resulted in a stagnated view that fails to acknowledge how different ways of knowing can shape the material world. Referring to communities with the authority to change design and practice on a large scale, he stated:

> I think, arguably the most important ingredient in these communities is an unwillingness or just a recognition that so much of this is the built world. These are human choices that humans made, and it's changeable. The disease state, maybe not, but everything that we build around it is. We made it this way and it doesn't have to be this way. It could be a different way.

Meaningfully, two informants involved in DIY were in medical professions (Aditi and Evelyn), two others were in training for such professions (Erica and Ramona), and several others had worked directly in research or other collaborations with medical professionals and commercial device manufacturers. So, while there was general consensus that the medical establishment fails to recognize lived experience in diabetes management, informants were actively working to address this gap, imagining a future medicine that values lived contributions.

The second transgression that underlies DIY experiences is the abandonment of the hegemonic perception of bodily risk for one that is more authentically rooted in disabled embodiment. Much like my informants who had received deep brain stimulation, whose understandings of invasiveness differed from those of their nondisabled physicians, DIY users made explicit that the ways in which they calculated risk were not the same as those employed by their nondisabled peers and regulatory bodies. Exemplified in Carolyn's assertion that "the disease is going to kill me if I don't do something," the calculations of people with T1D focused on the riskiness of continuing to use the stagnated strategies that had failed to achieve promised outcomes. In contrast, nondisabled people saw possible danger in new strategies for diabetes management. This differential understanding of risk is directly related to diverging experiences of embodiment. In other words, disabled embodiment serves as an epistemic resource for interpreting and acting on risk. As such, DIY users exemplify the recognition of embodiment as a source of unique social, political, and ontological knowledge. The shift away from cure to quality of life through a technological prosthetic exemplifies the power of embracing embodiment, especially nonnormative embodiment, as a source of expertise.

The final transgression that characterizes the DIY movement is the strong community ethos that resists and rejects the individualization key to medicalizing disability and chronic illness. The medicalization of disability, which recasts it as solely a biological phenomenon located exclusively within the body, relies on the identification and isolation of "maladaptive" bodies to maintain authority.

Privileging embodied and experiential knowledge is vital to the formation of a coherent DIY community. In many instances, building and using DIY technologies gives users an opportunity to assert the embodied and practical knowledge that had been invalidated or minimized in clinical settings, and thus to resist what feminist critical scholar Kristina Gupta describes as the process by which "medicine increases our reliance on medical experts and undermines our privileged relationship to our own bodies, while displacing alternative ways of understanding mind/body distress."[25] DIYAPS resembles what Phil Brown and colleagues call "embodied health movements." In these political formations, collective experience of illness serves as a "source of solidarity, motivation, and urgency."[26] Crucially, embodiment within embodied health movements serves as both an epistemic resource and a marker of credibility, in direct opposition to medical frameworks that favor professionalized knowledge over lived experience. These movements are distinguished from other social movements in that they insert and emphasize the physical bodymind, challenge hegemonic medical and scientific knowledge through knowledge produced by embodiment, and work with professionals to develop new methods of intervention. The first two characteristics in this list featured prominently in the interviews and guidance documents for DIYAPS, while the last was a source of tension for many informants, in part because of a perceived mismatch in priorities and understandings of diabetes between people with T1D and clinicians, technologists, and other professionals. However, as Melody said, "We don't necessarily have to work with companies, though we'd like to. We don't have to work with researchers, though we'd like to." The openness to consider these partnerships while not relying on the authority of perceived experts points to the boundary work carried out by DIY users, who not only rearticulate boundaries in formalized medicine to insert lived experience but also reimagine the types of knowledge and authority necessary at all.[27]

Rather than advocating for inviting embodied expertise into traditional scientific spaces, DIYAPS constructs a new space built on embodied expertise, with the option of inviting in traditionally marked scientific and medical experts. In this sense, DIYAPS has constructed a dispersed "cripspace," a space created by and for disabled people, privileging and celebrating disabled experience.[28] Rather than seeking assimilation into traditional medical and scientific spaces, DIY users construct a space with a different set of credibility politics built primarily on the assumption of embodied and experiential knowledge, albeit one that, as illustrated above, reproduces some of the knowledge politics found in clinical spaces. It is within this cripspace that generative possibilities emerge, not just in the technology but also in the reimagining of diabetes as a collective, collaborative experience.

Gender, Race, and Class in DIY Communities

While the majority of informants did not explicitly address intersectional experiences within DIYAPS communities, their comments were inflected with racialized, classed, and gendered experiences. Nearly all informants who disclosed their race identified as white, and all were highly educated, often with graduate-level education.[29] In terms of gender, the masculinized digital spaces that characterize open-source and hacking cultures are differentially experienced by women and femmes.[30] Generally speaking, fewer women are present in hacking communities than in other computing cultures, and these spaces typically reinscribe patriarchal paradigms, including meritocratic myths and sexist discourses.[31] Melody reflected on the significant frustration she experienced early on in DIYAPS spaces, feeling she was often ignored, dismissed, or mocked for her emphasis on communication and community building:

> This happened both physically in person as well as some of the comments and activity online. I think having a hundred percent male community and having the kind of community that was starting to replicate in the diabetes space wasn't necessarily a positive one, wasn't a welcoming one, and we certainly wouldn't be able to welcome larger contributors in the future. And I felt like that wasn't what we wanted for our community, so I kind of called it out.

Perhaps because of these early interventions, or because the DIYAPS movement resembles embodied health activism more closely than it resembles hacking communities, informants like Erica, who joined the community after it had been more firmly established, remarked on the distinct lack of the hacker archetype. Others like Aditi, however, referenced a still-present divide between "techie" and "non-techie" users. The "techies" were implied to be white, college-educated male-identifying coders in, as one set of DIY documentation suggested, "their darkened rooms" with their "creative and analytical brains," a characterization similar to Siân Brooke's articulation of hacker culture.[32] So, while DIY and open-source diabetes technology espouses an infinitely welcoming and infinitely collaborative discursive space, a distinct hierarchy is implied, with developers, often coded as male, above users, who are understood as more diverse. Several informants mentioned two particularly prominent women in the DIY community, usually in reference to their exceptional communication and interpersonal skills. These skills are tacitly feminine coded, and as such, as one informant noted, they tend to be perceived as less important. Yet informants again and again pointed to the accessible and welcoming tone in the DIY community as critical to their involvement.

Class also came into play in conversations about DIYAPS, particularly in regard to access to supplies, technology, and health literacy. This resonates with several recent reviews that have suggested that access to insulin pumps and CGMs is contingent on race and income level. In a U.S.-based study, Steven M. Willi and colleagues found that Black and Hispanic children with T1D were significantly less likely than their white counterparts to have insulin pumps.[33] In the United Kingdom, the Clinical Audit and Registries Management Service reported in 2016 that insulin pump use was significantly lower in regions experiencing socioeconomic deprivation.[34] Importantly, although the findings are less well understood, recent research suggests that clinicians have "strong yet often inaccurate views about individual patient capacity to use pumps successfully."[35] Perhaps such assumptions contribute to the image of the "advanced user" as educated, white, well-off, and compliant. While informants often discussed lack of access to technology, insulin insecurity, and insufficient health literacy as barriers to DIY, there was almost no explicit recognition of race or class in their constructions of the "advanced user" with both the requisite access and the self-responsibility to become a DIYAPS user. This absence raises questions about the potential invisibility of people of color, working-class people, people living in rural areas, and other marginalized groups in the DIYAPS community.

In this chapter, I have related the decision to pursue DIY technologies to the invalidation of user experience in traditional medical paradigms. In DIY communities, the celebration of individual experience and the perception of shared priorities create a culture of trust that is bolstered by a hacker ethic that promotes transparency, collaboration, and mutual support. DIYAPS offers a means of control over both diabetes and diabetes management—control that is often stripped away in more traditional settings. Informants also highlighted a differential risk calculus that leads them to view DIY as a viable choice, while those who are not engaged in day-to-day diabetes management see it as possibly dangerous. This divergence of perspectives points to the need for greater attentiveness to embodied and experiential expertise in the design of diabetes technologies and management practices. Finally, despite calls for universal access and acceptance, the interviews bring into focus a particular kind of person with T1D as the optimal user of DIY technologies, raising questions about who can and cannot contribute to and benefit from DIY systems.

Despite the communitarian approach that characterizes DIY spaces, an emphasis on self-responsibility—often cloaked in references to the engaged and advanced user—still permeates these communities, creating layers of stratification that may further marginalize already marginalized people with T1D. Tensions remain between messages of universal access and selective profiles of successful DIY users. Further, the value placed on self-governance and self-responsibility resonates with expectations produced under a neoliberal ableist paradigm. Even within the strong ethos of transparency and camaraderie that characterizes the DIY movement, users are still expected to shoulder the responsibility of management. DIYAPS is, after all, "doing an (n = 1) experiment," according to the guidance documents. Importantly, the parameters of self-governance in DIYAPS are not articulated by authority figures such as medical professionals or technologists; this distinguishes DIYAPS from the pressures of self-management as previously addressed in the literature.[36] Ultimately, while DIYAPS critically disrupts the hegemonic paradigm by shifting authority and credibility away from commercial medical devices, manufacturers, and clinicians and onto people managing diabetes, it also reinforces the neoliberal ableist paradigms of self-responsibility and body management.

Unlike the users of prenatal genetic screening and deep brain stimulation, who experience the double bind of personal accountability and epistemic invalidation, the DIYAPS community rejects the submissive patient role thrust on many with diabetes. Personal responsibility becomes communal obligation, or in Carolyn's words, the responsibility to "guard our own communities." The development of a coherent DIY community creates opportunities for alternative cultural imaginings about health, disability, and well-being.

In the Conclusion that follows, I draw together lessons from the three case studies presented in the preceding chapters to examine the necessity—and consequences—of knowledge, authority, and bodily transgressions in the pursuit of livable disabled lives. I move toward articulating a new embodied knowledge politic of medical technology rooted in the transformative, lifesaving, yet ultimately mundane transgressions that technology users must commit to survive the neoliberal ableist medical landscape.

Conclusion

Toward a New Embodied Knowledge Politic of Medical Technology

When I met Joel, he was in his mid-twenties, a PhD student working for a diabetes technology company on the West Coast of the United States. He'd been living with type 1 diabetes for more than a decade. The year before, he had built and started using a DIY artificial pancreas system. Prior to that, he had been frustrated with his care options and had tried to distance himself from all things diabetes. DIYAPS felt different, though. He found both a meaningful technological intervention and a community that shared and valued his experiences. He told me, "I'm not just beholden to whatever the medical companies say is appropriate, and whatever my endocrinologist, who doesn't actually want to get in depth with me, tells me to do, because I have this wealth of community knowledge that I can contribute to and draw from." The reciprocity and support he gained from the DIY community made any additional work or risk worthwhile. Of everyone I spoke to across all three cases, Joel expressed to me most succinctly how knowledge, accountability, and body management are inextricably linked. Of his choice to turn to DIY, he said:

> It's like the Matrix, when you take the pill and now you see how the world is, and you can do something about it, or you can just sit with it and not do anything with it. . . . I can't take away my knowledge and also take away my responsibility, I guess.

As I have demonstrated in the preceding chapters, user experiences of prenatal genetic screening and testing, deep brain stimulation, and DIYAPS reveal that human relationships to medical technology are both mundane and extraordinary, oppressive and liberating. In our current sociotechnical system, there is no way to exist in a nonnormative bodymind without transgressing the boundaries of medical authority or acceptable embodiment. Attempts to politicize disabled embodiment in the clinic are met with pressures to further individualize and privatize interventions, retrenching the authority of the medical establishment. Disabled people (or prospective parents of disabled people) are held personally accountable for ameliorating disability while their embodied, experiential, and practical expertise is invalidated in favor of clinical judgment or laboratory data. In other words, people are expected to manage, mitigate, or eliminate disability at the same time their experiences and choices are dismissed if they are in conflict with medical authority. The medical technologies my informants encountered simultaneously perpetuated and displaced neoliberal ableism, paradoxically reinforcing and alleviating personal responsibility and epistemic invalidation. They shaped discursive and material conditions by upholding hegemonic authority demanding closer approximation to the ideal bodymind, while displacing a small share of the everyday work of survival in an ableist world.

Medical technology users are imagining new social, political, and material arrangements both within and outside the clinic. In this Conclusion, I draw together insights from informants to sketch the characteristics of this new knowledge politic and its implications. I start by considering the role of autonomy and self-responsibility, arguing that neoliberal ableism acts as a driving force in the individualization, medicalization, and depoliticization of disability. To counteract this force, I imagine a less autonomous, less individualized subject in favor of a collective experience of disability. I then consider the necessary steps for taking embodied knowledge seriously, which include excavating the biases that continually cast disabled life as undesirable and low quality. Next, I characterize informants' transgressions across the boundaries defining bodily integrity and knowledge authority committed in pursuit of agency within the medical establishment and call for a reimagining of these boundaries. Finally, I consider the ambivalent role of technology itself. I do not include prescriptive recommendations for the adoption or rejection of any of the medical technologies examined here; rather, I point out the need to make explicit the social and political complexities that frame and contextualize the individual and communal experience of pursuing medical care.

This suggestion challenges both techno-optimistic discourses of hegemonic science and the techno-pessimistic stance that characterizes critical studies of technology, embracing a more pedestrian relationship between bodyminds and technology. I close with a call to redirect our technoscientific energies away from managing and mitigating disabled bodyminds and toward abolishing neoliberal ableism.

Forging a Less Autonomous Subject

Responsibility—for disability management, toward future generations, as an aspect of citizenship—was central to informants' articulation of their experiences with medical technology. For many, responsibility meant an obligation to meet prescribed clinical outcomes and inevitable blame when one fell short. Clinicians chastised people with T1D for poor control of their blood sugar. Pregnant people stewed over potentially preventable prenatal conditions. DBS implantees had outcomes that did not match their own or others' expectations. In this particular iteration of responsibility, a clinician—or, more likely, a set of clinical tools—determined both the mode of measurement and the standard by which the individual was judged. Informants were labeled as "out of range," "high risk," or otherwise anomalous. Bodies became standardized in ways that did not reflect their ambiguity and uncertainty, and informants were blamed for subsequently failing to meet detached, clinical standards—standards that, as Gary pointed out regarding clinical guidelines for A1C, may not even be achievable. In other words, responsibility demands the pursuit of the idealized nondisabled bodymind. All other embodiment is unacceptable. Existing as disabled—or carrying a potential future disabled bodymind—constitutes a de facto failure. This type of responsibility relies on the tacit acceptance of clinical markers of health as synonymous with ideal embodiment. The authority to categorize and delineate acceptable embodiment falls within the purview of medicine, while the responsibility to attain and maintain it falls squarely on the individual.

Under neoliberalism, human experience is individualized. Each person is expected to act autonomously, to self-regulate in line with social mores and practices, and to do work that is legible to the state and market. This context immediately subjects disabled people to scrutiny, judgment, and discrimination.[1] Across all three cases, the perceived inferiority of disabled bodyminds that pervades social and political life translated into feelings of guilt, shame, and self-blame for signifiers of difference. Such guilt, in concert with the demands on the neoliberal subject to self-manage, creates a context in which medical intervention to identify and eliminate disability seems both natural and necessary. For some informants who received prenatal genetic testing, there was a preemptive guilt at the thought of birthing a disabled child. As a pregnant Rosalie voiced, "If something is wrong with the baby, it's my fault." Informants who received deep brain stimulation and those using do-it-yourself artificial pancreas systems reported feelings of shame related to the observable differences linked to their disabilities. Lynn lauded DBS as alleviating the shame associated with the facets of her Parkinson's, like tremor, that were "obvious to people." In the DIYAPS case, several informants spoke of recognition of difference from their peers without diabetes as an unwanted rite of passage during youth. As Erica recalled about her teenage years, "I didn't want to be different." Disablement, for many informants, was inflected with feelings of alienation, isolation, and judgment from others. This affective experience is relevant both because it is instrumental in prompting individuals to pursue medical intervention and because it expands the clinical understanding of disability beyond discrete, measurable, physiological symptoms. When disability is related to difference, and difference to shame, the ideal normate becomes reinscribed as the only desirable or valuable person.[2] Medical interventions to ameliorate difference are naturalized as both logical and appealing when shame is internalized.

However, neoliberalism dictates that an individual's medical decisions to intervene on the disabled bodymind (or to detect future disability through genetic screening and testing) benefit not just the individual but also the public. By preventing, treating, or curing disability, a person moves toward the ideal of the productive citizen. Disability is intrinsically linked to nonproductivity. As Mateo Pimentel and I have written elsewhere, the ability/disability binary in contemporary Western societies is articulated through narratives of capitalist productivity: "What an 'able bodymind' is *able* to do is implicit; such a bodymind is capable of joining the labor market, capable of being efficient, . . . capable of turning a profit for themselves, or more likely, for their employer. Any bodymind that does not meet such criteria is thus considered 'disabled.'"[3] Confirming this perspective, informants interpreted responsibility as maintaining or regaining independence and economic productivity in the face of disabled embodiment. As John stated, his decision to pursue DBS was informed by his desire to have "less dependence on others." Throughout the cases examined in this study, informants noted that medical technologies enabled access to self-responsibility, productivity, and independence—all neoliberal ideals. For those receiving prenatal genetic screening and testing, for example, technological intervention during pregnancy was a signifier of responsible parenthood and, by extension, responsible citizenship. For those receiving DBS, surgery opened up a pathway to return to previous economic productivity and reliability, regardless of whether that came to fruition. Intervention, particularly curative intervention where possible, becomes an expectation in the pursuit of moral and responsible citizenship. The assumption that all users are equally able to choose or reject medical technologies freely, independently, and in the absence of external pressures "obscures the complex histories, webs, and attachments of technoscience," as Alison Kafer writes.[4]

As Inga Bostad and Halvor Hanisch argue, reconceptualizing freedom to include expressions of inter/dependence and the individual subject to account for human variation can yield a significantly different understanding of disability. Rather than beginning with an assumption about who is the ideal and free subject, they suggest employing an "inductive modesty" that recognizes that "to accept difference—that which is unknown to me—is to accept that some aspects of life (both the lives of others and one's own life) will remain unknown."[5] The narrow understanding of acceptable embodiment that colors perceptions of personal responsibility excludes experiences of disability that do not demand medical intervention. Informants, however, brought with them expanded understandings of responsibility that opened up space to reconsider both the nature of disability and collective knowledge about disability management.

The individualization of medical intervention serves to depoliticize disabled embodiment, foreclosing on futures rooted in collective liberation.[6] As Kafer observes, "When disability has been placed solely in the medical framework, and both disability and the medical world are portrayed as apolitical, then disability has no place in radical politics and social movements—except as a problem to be eradicated."[7] Such depoliticization fractures solidarity, reinforcing hierarchical understandings of disabled embodiment. For example, the users of medical technologies in the cases presented here often shared their judgments of others who made different choices or had different outcomes after selecting or rejecting medical technology. While informants across all three cases expressed openness and nonjudgmental attitudes toward how others live with disability (or the potential for disability), many simultaneously expressed disapproval of those whose practices did not align with their own. These informants frequently perceived others as not being responsible or accountable for themselves or their prospective children, where "responsible" typically meant self-educated, self-motivated, and self-governing. Such judgments allowed them to identify others with similar conditions not as their peers but as people in need of support and guidance.

While this particular facet of responsibility may be interpreted as the internalization of neoliberal ableist discourses, an alternative explanation—rooted in shared experiences of ableism—is possible. Throughout all three cases, informants explicitly recognized the biased and discriminatory systems in which they were enmeshed, and what I have identified as judgment may in fact be read as a form of protective guidance. In other words, informants often acknowledged the power of passing as nondisabled through medical interventions as a way to circumvent stigma, and they wanted to provide guidance so that others would not have the same discriminatory, invalidating experiences they themselves encountered. While some scholars have strongly critiqued passing as nondisabled as a "reinforcement of hegemonic power," others have noted that it is also an act of self-protection against the stigma, discrimination, and violence regularly enacted against disabled people. Peta Cox, for example, acknowledges the legitimacy of passing as self-protection rather than denial of identity, noting that for people with mental illness, the "costs of not passing can be quite high," so avoiding them through the "deliberate and strategic performance" of passing is justified.[8] Viewing the adoption of medical technologies as a form of passing as nondisabled—or at least as approximating the absence of disability—casts expressions of judgment toward nonadopters in a different light. In both the DBS and DIYAPS cases, nearly all informants' statements of judgment were paired with expressions of altruism toward others experiencing similar circumstances. Perhaps the clearest argument for this alternative explanation appeared in the DIYAPS case, with Evelyn's statement, "I think a lot of us have a really strong desire to make the person coming after us's road a little easier than the road we had, because we all had different struggles, but struggles." Many users of DIYAPS technologies shared that they had acute feelings of personal responsibility for their health and safety, which they linked directly to what they viewed as the failure of clinicians and device manufacturers to provide the support they needed. But, as Evelyn's remark illustrates, the responsibility that informants felt toward the community of DIYers (and people with T1D more generally) also galvanized them to contribute to DIY technologies and community. This example directly resists the neoliberal value of individualization. Additionally, while many informants acknowledged past difficulties related to accepting their difference from their nondisabled peers, almost universally, they had taken up diabetes as a social and political identity, and thus resisted the subordination of disabled bodyminds. Echoes of these sentiments can be found in the interviews of DBS informants who contributed to support groups, and, to a lesser extent, those of prospective parents who turned to online pregnancy forums with their questions and concerns.

For informants who were either prospective parents, as in the case of PGT, or current guardians of children with diabetes, as in the DIYAPS case, individual responsibility extended into responsibility toward future generations. For Abby, the decision to receive prenatal genetic screening during her pregnancy was in part motivated by a desire to provide her future child the best health care upon birth. "You're not going to stay at your same doctor," she told me, "and get treated the same way if your child has [a genetic condition]." Genetic counselor Theresa acknowledged the difference in feelings of accountability in seeking medical care for oneself versus one's future child, saying of prospective parents, "They feel obligated, because of course you have to do what's best 'cause it's your unborn baby." The guardians of young children with T1D noted a similar distinction. While recognizing the "sheer between my experience as a parent caring for a child and the experience of someone who actually lives with the disease," as Gordon stated, these guardians also often expressed an enormous feeling of responsibility to give their children the best possible chance for a good quality of life. Several informants suggested that this feeling of parental responsibility is in part what enables the DIY community to thrive. Erica, who herself has diabetes, referred to one prominent member of the DIY community as being particularly effective in part because of her role as a parent:

> I just always remind her of how much, really what she's done for the community by building out these docs and making it so easy to understand what you did and how to do it for yourself and your kids. Like, her desire was to give moms the information to better their kids' lives—because she knew if anyone was going to do it, it was going to be a diabetic mom.

While informants in the DIYAPS case explicitly acknowledged that guardianship does not equate with embodied experience of T1D, those in the PGT case did not discuss any comparable difference. The liminality of pregnancy and the abstraction of the future disabled child obscures the distinction between the embodiment of the PGT user and the disabled embodiment of a potential future child. Although beyond the scope of my analysis, the tensions between perceived parental responsibility toward (actual and potential) disabled children and the need to weigh the experiential expertise of nondisabled caregivers against the embodied knowledge of disabled people warrant deeper consideration.

Haunting all of these facets of responsibility is the specter of the independent individual subject as free and endlessly autonomous. When individual freedom is highly valued and equated with independence, any dependence that arises from disablement is interpreted as an impediment to full personhood. Arseli Dokumacı compellingly argues that the unique and essential knowledge of disabled embodiment emerges not from endless possibility but from the constraints of navigating "the least hospitable, least welcoming, and the least permitting of circumstances."[9] Embodied knowledge, then, depends not on our limitless autonomy but on our ability to adapt and to imagine accommodating futures into being within a constrained present. The mythical limitlessly autonomous figure obfuscates the factors that inequitably constrain our agency. Further, as Kafer argues, "this focus on personal responsibility precludes any discussion on social, political, or collective responsibility."[10]

Systems of oppression continue to disenfranchise and enact harm on disabled bodyminds, coercing all of us to embody—to whatever extent possible—a nondisabled ideal. Under this regime, voluntary, autonomous informed consent is an impossible standard to meet, in the clinic or anywhere else. Failure to address the ableism and disableism that pervade medical and social cultures, especially the inequitable pressures that come to bear on nonnormative bodyminds, risks perpetuating them in design and practice. To move toward a new embodied knowledge politic, then, first requires a reimagining of the subject as both less autonomous and less individual than the neoliberal ableist narrative would have us believe. Such a shift immediately relieves the pressures of responsibility and accountability predicated on the assumptions that a medical technology user has boundless autonomy to pursue ideal embodiment and that there is consensus regarding what that embodiment can and should be. This requires recognition of the social, political, and material constraints that both produce and contribute to disability and that limit individual autonomy. Second, we must move beyond individualized narratives that cast medical technology users as isolated autonomous subjects within medical systems and turn toward a collective or coalitional politic. Such a reenvisioning resists depoliticization, further eroding medicine's individualizing power and encouraging greater solidarity.

Making Embodied Knowledge Credible

The meaning of disability is constantly in flux. Cultural, social, and political frameworks influence how and when bodily difference becomes disability. Medical categorization is not a neutral observation of a natural world but a political act that is historically, geographically, and socially contingent.[11] Because disability constitutes an unstable category, its ontological, social, and political meanings shift along with the discourse around and use of medical technologies. Medical interventions become possible only through the standardization and categorization of disabled bodyminds, which can occur only through credible knowledge production about what disability is and who is responsible for managing it.

According to sociologist Peter Conrad, the professionalization of medicine took place in modernity in part as the result of a need to fill an authority vacuum caused by the secularization of Western society.[12] Medical categories, diagnoses, and authority have since been used as means of social control, particularly over populations deemed undesirable. Beyond that, as Susan Wendell asserts, medical authority has gained the power to determine what is ontologically, socially, and politically real through the pathologization and subordination of disabled and otherwise nonnormative embodiments.[13] In this way, medical knowledge and authority are intrinsically linked. Transgressions of this knowledge and authority are committed when individuals occupying the patient role gain too much knowledge or control over their bodyminds, disrupting and supplanting medical authority.

Therefore, the attempt to relocate credible knowledge about disability to nonmedical contexts is destabilizing to a medical establishment that seeks to control the naming, location, and management of disability. Perceived transgressions of authority occur most often when disability is disrupted as a biologically discrete category and relocated to practical and experiential contexts. The datafication and visualization of disability through karyotypes, MRIs, and A1C values tacitly support an understanding of disability as a purely biological phenomenon. Additionally, the measurement and visualization of disability, in whatever form, are commonly used as means of bolstering trust in clinical authority. For example, in the case of DBS, visualization tools such as MRI scans allow users to see the precise areas of their brains to be intervened on, which helps them develop trust toward their clinicians. Disability becomes tangible through visualization while simultaneously remaining fully and firmly inside medicine's jurisdiction.

Further, framing disability as a physiological feature rather than an identity retrenches the Cartesian duality of mind and body. As DBS recipient Fred stated of Parkinson's disease, "You fight your own body. You have to do things when your body is telling you not to." This duality delegitimates embodiment as a valid form of knowledge by severing person from body. In the case of PGT, clinicians largely emphasized the perceived realness of biological and physiological dimensions of chromosomal difference—as opposed to the social impacts—despite recognizing prospective parents' desire for lived knowledge of disability. Genetic counselor Anton, for example, stated that biological outcomes were more "tangible," and Marcie said, "We [genetic counselors] usually start with the medical—mostly because it's easier. And it's a—it doesn't lead to other discussions." Combined with the perceived animosity between genetic counselors and disabled communities, this hard line serves to further essentialize disability to its genetic and physiological components and to restrict prospective parents from access to embodied knowledge from disabled people, knowledge that could provide essential context for informed consent.

Key to relocating the power to name and manage disability is establishing credibility to speak about it authoritatively. As discussed in chapter 1, medicalization has allowed for the creep of clinical authority into all areas of life. Enabled through professionalization with strictly regulated access to who can obtain membership, medical authority has established seemingly inflexible boundaries between agential actors and passive subjects. Perceptions of inflexibility bled through in interviews across case studies even as informants recognized and promoted the value of experiential and embodied knowledge, suggesting an awareness of the power differentials that characterize medicalization. For example, Barry, the husband of DBS user Mary, flatly stated that his wife could not offer other DBS recipients advice because "she's not a doctor. You can't say anything." Gordon, the father of a young user of DIYAPS technologies, conceded that "cure is so inaccessible" when discussing the future of DIY diabetes technology, continuing, "Like it's the specialized guild and priesthood of medicine that has all these boundaries around it that you can't cross." Marcie, a genetic counselor, spoke about the seemingly obligatory nature of prenatal genetic testing and alluded to the implicit pressures faced by prospective parents: "Why would you say no to your doctor?" Each of these examples, in the midst of a broader discussion uplifting lived experience, points to a recognition of systems of power that continually deny authority to nonprofessionals.

The policing of knowledge within the clinic often forces users of medical technologies to look outside the clinic for information, an act that produces increased tension in clinical interactions. Clinicians may view users' external research as evidence of a lack of trust in their medical expertise.[14] A study of people seeking rheumatology care, for example, found that those who did their own research online feared being perceived as challenging, noncompliant, or confrontational.[15] These findings resonate with the experiences of informants who used DIYAPS technologies, who, judging from their interactions with medical professionals and manufacturers, interpreted their knowledge and practice as threatening to the authority of specialists and commercial developers. As Evelyn stated of the commercial response to DIY: "Instead of viewing it as an opportunity, they view it as a threat. They view it as competition and not cooperation." Further, as discussed in chapter 1, beyond the deprioritization of lay knowledge in the clinic generally, disabled people face a particular and acute epistemic invalidation of their knowledge, especially knowledge about their own lives.[16] In other words, assumptions about the unworthiness, undesirability, and poor quality of disabled lives often shut disabled people out of these narratives completely.

Informants were able to establish credibility in some cases by recognizing and working with the systems of authority that had previously denied them. DBS user Mary, for example, formed personal and professional relationships with neurosurgeons and other medical practitioners, leveraging her proximity to medical authority to present herself to her medical team as a credible source. The DIYAPS community deploys technical and scientific language and processes around experimentation, scientific inquiry, and medical risk, and movement leaders frequently attend academic and medical conferences. This latter example brings to mind Steven Epstein's account of "activist-experts" during the HIV/AIDS crisis, whose acquisition of scientific knowledge and use of jargon gained them sufficient credibility in the eyes of the federal government that they were allowed to participate in the oversight process for drug trials.[17] Like those activists, in taking this approach the DIYAPS community in some ways implicitly endorses the hegemonic method of scientific inquiry and authority, potentially eroding its members' contributions as embodied and experiential knowers. This may help to explain the implicit inclusion criteria for who can participate in DIYAPS: financially stable, self-motivated, well educated. On the other hand, as noted in chapter 4, the DIY diabetes community has cohered around a social and political identity rather than a medical category—specifically in their identification with and affinity for broader disability communities—signaling a movement away from clinical authority and medicalization.

Mismatches in priorities, expectations, and lived experience have profound consequences for clinical interactions. First, the nature and amount of information that prospective users desire is profoundly disconnected from the information clinicians believe they are obligated to provide. Second, both micro- and macro-level transformations are needed to address epistemic invalidation in clinical interactions. Experiences of invalidation cannot be remedied through increased attentiveness to individual context alone. Transformation requires a rearticulation of knowledge and authority in medicine that accounts for the embodied and experiential expertise of disabled people. Kristi Kirschner and Raymond Curry assert the vital importance of disability-related competencies for physicians. They call for a restructuring of care to center the patient, such that the clinician is responsive to the individual's perceptions of quality of life, rather than to the clinician's own assumptions made in the absence of lived experience.[18] As this project has demonstrated, the lack of appreciation and tolerance for a quality of life that varies from the rigidly independent nondisabled ideal has significant impacts on people's perceptions of themselves and their choices around medical technologies. Lisa Iezzoni and Linda Long-Bellil suggest that even well-intentioned clinicians cannot and should not develop training and practices for disability-related health care in the absence of disabled people, in part because clinicians "'just don't get' important aspects of the lives and expectations of persons with disabilities."[19] Pathways forward include the introduction of disabled people as medical educators during the training of clinicians. For example, it is becoming increasingly common for disabled people to be invited to participate as "standardized patients," volunteers who are trained to work with medical students in simulated clinical environments.[20] Further, as suggested by several informants across case studies in this project, clear and formal access to resources in the community, such as other people who have confronted the same kinds of decisions around medical intervention, could provide crucial support. Additionally, diverse perspectives must be represented in the organizational and regulatory bodies that animate and articulate visions for medical design and practice. Diversity should be cultivated in political roles, given the relationship between technological progress and American social values, as well as in leadership and advisory positions within professional organizations, hospital systems, and regulatory bodies. The introduction of new technologies into health care systems transforms the choices and consequences for everyone, not just prospective users. Involving disabled people, with their embodied and experiential expertise, in the design, practice, and regulation of these technologies, rather than only as passive recipients, could crucially transform both how people experience medical technologies and what medical technologies enter the market.

Assertions of embodied and practical expertise trouble the medical establishment's ostensible control over current and future disabled bodyminds. In a political and social environment that grants that establishment authority over embodiment, such assertions are viewed as transgressions. They challenge hegemonic narratives of disabled lives as always tragic, undesirable, and in need of elimination, subverting expected regimes of knowledge production. Many of the informants I spoke with knowingly transgressed these boundaries, advocating for the generative possibilities of embodiment as expertise. In such resistance, as Dan Goodley writes, "being disabled is not a tragedy but a possibility, an affirmation, a queer or crip space for rethinking what it means to be human, to live a quality life, and a life with quality."[21] This transformation requires not just inviting disabled perspectives but conducting a collective excavation of our cultural understanding of what makes a good life and what does not. To embrace disabled alternative imaginaries, we must take seriously the embodied knowledge of disabled people, listening to disabled people and believing what they have to say.

Redrawing Boundaries

Conflicts arise between medical technology users and clinicians, device manufacturers, regulators, family members, and community members when users commit perceived transgressions across the boundaries of "acceptable" embodiment and disability management. In this section, I explore two interconnected types of transgressions: those related to bodily integrity and those related to knowledge acquisition. How and by whom these boundaries are drawn and surveilled reveals a fundamental power imbalance between medical technology users and the medical establishment. As users of these technologies are not in positions of authority to determine the boundaries, they are viewed as the transgressors.

Their transgressions signal a shifting away from the passive and receptive patient role into the role of agential actor, which often simultaneously challenges the pathologization of nonnormative bodyminds. By destabilizing the professional–patient relationship, users blur the "boundaries as to who does the curing (and, ipso facto, decides and designs the treatment regimen) and who needs curing (or who receives the treatment)."[22]

Within Western medicine, the preservation or restoration of the nondisabled body is taken for granted as the end goal of medical intervention. The invisibility of ableism in this medical discourse means that conflicts about the desirability and worth of bodily interventions abound without a critical framework to interrogate them. Nondisabled clinicians understand approaches to medicine that preserve bodily integrity to be common sense.[23] Disabled embodiment contributes to a meaning of risk and bodily integrity that runs counter to this nondisabled hegemonic interpretation. When medical technology users bring with them a different understanding of how and when bodily integrity is violated—and therefore a different understanding of acceptable risk—they challenge clinical authority. In both the DBS and DIYAPS cases, users had typically been living with and managing chronic illness and disability for years prior to engaging with these technologies. For prospective parents pursuing PGT, these transgressions were more abstract, rooted in ideas about what kinds of future children are acceptable to bring into the world.

As discussed in chapter 3, DBS is often presented to prospective users as a "last resort" technology, owing to the physically invasive nature of implantation. However, as Bradley noted about his experiences with narcotics prior to receiving DBS, "your body's not being cut open, but it's so invasive in your life in so many other facets." He and others highlighted that medication regimens, which typically precede surgical intervention, led to surveillance, stigma, and side effects that they perceived as more invasive than implantation. The framing of DBS as significantly more invasive, and therefore often withheld until a number of other potential interventions are attempted first, reveals a narrow perspective that fails to account for a person's life outside the clinic. Further, DBS and many other technologically dependent medical interventions contain a paradox regarding bodily autonomy. While DBS is often positioned as necessary for reclaiming independence and autonomy, as John Gardner and Narelle Warren point out, "for such devices to work correctly, users are required to be tethered to specialist clinical teams, and hence, their autonomy depend[s] on a network of relations of care."[24] This dependent-independence is further complicated by the commonplace violation of disabled bodyminds in medical contexts, often framed as being in the disabled people's best interest. Enduring what Mia Mingus describes as "forced intimacy," disabled people are often subjected to nonconsensual touch and invasive questioning, all while being expected to perform emotional labor within medical contexts.[25] A failure to account for the complex networks of dependencies produced by any medical intervention results in strained clinical communication when users and clinicians have competing—and often invisibilized—priorities and expectations.

Relatedly, disabled technology users face additional scrutiny for taking risks that nondisabled people may perceive as jeopardizing their health and bodyminds. In the case of DIYAPS, nondisabled clinicians and family members expressed more fears and concerns about DIY technologies than users did, because they failed to grasp the burden of risk, uncertainty, and decision-making that accompanies the everyday engagement of chronic illness. According to users, nondisabled others interpreted DIYAPS as transgressing bodily integrity by risking the users' health, while the users observed little difference between DIY and the daily risks of self-management. Carolyn, for example, shared, "I didn't have any anxiety or any fear. My [nondiabetic] husband did. 'How do you know this isn't going to kill you?' And I think my answer might have been, 'Well, the disease is going to kill me if I don't do something.'" Both the DBS and DIYAPS cases reveal differential understandings of risk and embodiment. For those who are not disabled or not actively engaging with disability on a daily basis, the wholeness and incorruptibility of the bodymind is taken for granted. Transgressing the boundaries of the body, through either surgical intervention or off-label treatments, pollutes the pure and ideal bodymind. For disabled people, who embody risk daily and who have been subjected to scrutiny, violation, and transgression at the hands of the medical establishment, issues of risk and invasiveness are weighed differently.

The preservation of bodily integrity also sits at the heart of the development and use of PGT. As Ruth Hubbard writes, the use of

PGT to identify certain genetic conditions assumed to be undesirable allows technology companies and clinicians to answer the question "Who should and who should not inhabit the world?" in the absence of those they discuss.[26] By the time prospective parents encounter PGT in the clinic, the delineation between allowable and disallowable bodily differences has been cemented so thoroughly that it is rarely challenged. The transgression here, then, is the continued existence of disabled people who might otherwise have been screened out. As Marsha Saxton writes, "Many of us with disabilities might have been prenatally screened and aborted if tests had been available to our mothers. I've actually heard people say, 'Too bad that baby with [*x* disease] didn't "get caught" in prenatal screening.'"[27] What follows from the construction of the disabled bodymind as a violation of bodily integrity is the absence of embodied disability from the prenatal clinic altogether.

The second, and related, type of transgression includes those that crossed perceived acceptable thresholds of knowledge acquisition. For prospective parents receiving prenatal genetic testing, there was a limit—albeit an ill-defined one—to how much knowledge about a future child's genetic makeup was imperative for them to have in order to perform responsible parenthood; any knowledge beyond that limit was unnecessary or even risky. The appropriate level of knowledge, in these cases, was synonymous with the recommendation of a health care professional. Wishing to know more—for example, through screening for a genetic condition that the future child was not particularly at risk for—was construed as an impediment to responsible parenthood. Clinicians assumed that "too much" information would create anxiety or confusion, clouding prospective parents' judgment. As Melanie recalled, a clinician warned her against a full panel genetic screening by saying, "Be careful with that one. . . . You do that you're going to find something." How some genetic conditions, such as Down syndrome and trisomies 13 and 18, become defined as necessary to know about prior to birth, while others—nebulously described by Melanie's clinician as "something"—do not, remains firmly within the purview of medical professionals. This knowledge conflict highlights a broader disjunction between what clinicians perceive as useful or necessary information and what prospective parents need or desire to know. Richard Street Jr. and Paul Haidet found a similar mismatch when they compared physicians' perceptions of their patients' beliefs and values with how the patients themselves described those values. In general, physicians were very poor judges of their patients' health beliefs, tending to assume they were more closely aligned with their own than they actually were.[28] Prospective parent Abby provided an example of the frustration that arises from the gatekeeping of knowledge in the clinic. She recalled being denied access to information about fertility treatments even though she directly requested it: "[My clinician] was like, 'Oh we won't even talk about that now.' . . . It's like why can't I? Like why can't I talk about it? It'd be better if I talked about it with you than if I Googled it. So, like, why not?"

Across cases, a hierarchy of authority was evident. Users' authoritative claims rooted in embodiment or experience were often dismissed or invalidated by clinicians in the face of conflicting laboratory or clinical knowledge. Recipients of DBS in particular expressed personal value in the practical and embodied expertise of disability but experienced dismissal of that knowledge by medical professionals. This disconnect eroded clinical trust and contributed to the formation of oppositional relationships. Vickie's conflict with her DBS care team over adjusting and eventually removing her DBS exemplified this pattern. She stated, "They did what they wanted, and they weren't listening to me to be honest with you." While others spoke of similar strained relationships, phrases such as "but I'm not a doctor" inflected their remarks with a resignation about the power of medical authority. Such divisions appear not only in the clinic but also in the design of medical devices themselves, signaling a distance from lived experience in all aspects of medical authority.

As discussed above, authority also stemmed from the ability to quantify or visualize biological aspects of disability, a process typically controlled by clinicians. In DIYAPS spaces, however, knowledge of and ownership over data became a means of empowerment as well as a source of information to share within the community. Such strategies have long served marginalized people resisting hostile medicalization. For example, Michelle Murphy writes about the reclamation of bodily autonomy through the careful and communal observation of one's own body among participants of the Menstrual Cycle Study of 1975.[29] In this study, which emerged from the feminist self-help movement, nine women undertook an extensive series of daily measurements and observations via vaginal self-exam. Rather than seeking to standardize an understanding of the menstrual cycle, the participants asserted the complexity and diversity of reproductive biology and the knowledge that can be attained only through careful daily observation.[30] The adoption and adaptation of medical technoscience were central to this study, as they have been for DIYAPS. By accessing the data from her continuous glucose monitor while attempting to make an alarm that would wake her out of sleep in the event of low blood sugar, Dana Lewis unlocked the possibility of closing the loop for DIYAPS users. Gabi Schaffzin, a disabled scholar, provides an additional example through the co-option of data produced by his Fitbit and 23andMe profile into an artistic project, rejecting the medicalization, datafication, and objectification of his disabled bodymind for profit.[31] These examples nuance interpretations of technologies that datafy the body, demonstrating that they can serve as sources of power rather than oppression.

The experiences of DIYAPS users further illustrate how awareness of the medical establishment's authority and distance breeds resentment, dissatisfaction, and action. Because of the collective nature of the DIY diabetes community, the knowledge and authority transgressions of the "rogue cowboy hackers" were not discrete moments of clinical interaction but a calculated form of resistance against a medical authority that refused to recognize the experiential knowledge of the T1D community. DIYAPS directly resists the submissive patient role, in which a person with T1D quietly and gratefully accepts the guidance of the professional. This form of resistance explicitly rejects the authority of a detached medical establishment, calling out its distance from the lived realities of disability. Ultimately, the fissures between embodied experience and medical authority necessitate the above-articulated transgressions. Users of these technologies are caught in an impossible standard in which they are expected to acquire a certain amount of knowledge in order to be perceived as responsible, self-contained neoliberal subjects, but are condemned as reckless, threatening, or dangerous if they pursue too much knowledge or control over their bodyminds. A new embodied knowledge politic of medical technology requires reimagining the boundaries of acceptable bodyminds and knowledge acquisition.

The Mundanity of Technology

This book, as I say in the Introduction, is both about and not about medical technology. My proposed embodied knowledge politic is likewise both about and not about medical technology. I offer no prescriptive remedies, nor do I recommend wholesale adoption or rejection of any category of technological intervention. None of the technologies described in this text are extraordinary in their design or use, or in the constraints and opportunities they produce. We are constantly inundated with messages of techno-optimism that articulate medical technology as a form of salvation from our unpredictable embodiment. In response, critical disability studies and feminist science and technology studies have consistently condemned and critiqued medical technologies as extensions of regimes of power subordinating marginalized people. The personal accounts collected in this book, however, challenge both of these perspectives. Informants struck a decidedly ambivalent note about their relationships with technology. The technologies examined here are neither wholly liberatory nor wholly subordinating, troubling the techno-determinism that animates most discourses of technology and disability. Rather, engagement between bodyminds and technologies is something far more plebeian. As Abene, a thirty-five-year-old DIYAPS user from Spain, stated after sharing the relief she felt upon using this new system, "It has changed the way I live with my illness, but it has not changed me as a person." Regrounding the experience of medical technology in everyday experience unravels the alluring rhetoric of technological transformation. This balance is reminiscent of Mallory Kay Nelson, Ashley Shew, and Bethany Stevens's meditation on their personal relationships with technology as disabled women. They do not condemn or endorse any specific technological relationship, instead appreciating the uncertain possibilities of disabled bodyminds entwined with technology. "There is no one right way to be disabled," they write, "nor is there one right way to negotiate one's body in the world with technologies. There isn't even one technology that counts as a solution. None of this is super: it is all everyday."[32]

For the individual users in the cases examined in this book, the curative promise of medical technologies, even in the preventive sense of prenatal genetic testing, was not of much significance. What mattered far more were the impacts of the technologies on day-to-day life, which were substantially distanced from the discrete and rigid diagnostic and symptomatic measurements of the clinic. In the case of PGT, prospective parents often expressed being comforted by the knowledge they gained to prepare for an upcoming birth. With DBS, the impacts users mentioned included the ability to make adjustments at home using a patient remote. For DIYAPS users, the practical impacts of the technology encompassed such things as being able to get a full night's sleep without catastrophic blood sugar lows and the ability to monitor a young child's blood sugar from hundreds of miles away. In all cases, informants spoke about what mattered in their lives, lives that extended far beyond clinical markers of health and illness.

In my analysis, I was especially struck by a shared benefit across cases that had little to do with what the technologies were designed to detect, mitigate, or prevent. In the face of the burden of neoliberal individual responsibility, the adoption of medical technology became a method by which to displace the cognitive and emotional burden of navigating a neoliberal ableist world with a nonnormative bodymind—or with the potential to create one. For example, by transferring the immediate choices of diabetes management to an algorithm in DIYAPS, the user also displaces some of the daily burden of body management. By utilizing DBS to reduce tremor, a person with Parkinson's can mitigate the affective impacts of navigating the world in a visibly disabled bodymind. By screening for and diagnosing genetic differences in the fetus, potential parents distance and guard themselves from future stigma and judgment.

Stephen Horrocks makes a similar argument about the datafication and technification of diabetes management through commercial technologies such as insulin pumps and continuous glucose monitors. He reflects on the desire for cure expressed by many with diabetes, writing that "the desire for a post-Diabetic life—so often actually conceptualized as a pre-Diabetic life—is in many ways a desire to escape the labor and torque characteristic of life with a chronic illness. In practice, the desire is discursively linked to a desire for the experience of able-bodiedness in an able-bodied world, a desire to feel normal."[33] Medical technologies, then, are not simply interventions on biological difference—they are also tools for alleviating the social and political burden of being disabled in an ableist world. However, designers of medical technologies rarely call on lived experience, and so design often falls short of user desires. "They just don't think like a patient thinks," Mary, a DBS user, remarked when discussing a new design for a DBS patient remote that would be unusable for anyone with dexterity issues. She and her husband, Barry, suggested that people with Parkinson's should be designing and developing these tools to avoid such gross mismatches between bodymind and environment. Contextual, embodied, and practical knowledge grants insight into the material-discursive world that, as evidenced by the many examples of "bad design" raised here and elsewhere, is absent from much of medical device design.

Throughout the cases I analyzed, informants expressed frustration with, distrust in, and dismissal of commercial medical technologies in part because their designs fail to acknowledge, account for, or incorporate the daily lives of the people who use them. Rather, as they emerge from a hegemonic, positivist scientific framework, they perpetuate and proliferate bias, be that the androcentrism that casts prospective parents as "moral pioneers," to borrow Rayna Rapp's term, or the ableism that bars many people with T1D from accessing their data to manage their own care. Privileging the standpoints of nonscientists who live with medical technologies reveals a deep fissure sustained by the systemic exclusion of lived experience from the design and deployment of these technologies.

Generative alternatives exist, however, in subaltern spaces such as the DIYAPS community. In these contexts, "the lived experience of disability," Aimi Hamraie and Kelly Fritsch write, "creates specific expertise and knowledge that informs technoscientific practice."[34] While many DIYAPS users still subscribe to ideals of personal responsibility and accountability, the development of a coherent DIY community has created an opportunity for alternative cultural imaginings about health, disability, and well-being. To again call on M. Remi Yergeau's concept of criptastic hacking, such spaces "[rail] against forced normalization, one that moves from body-tweaking to something collective, activist, and systemic."[35] While DIYAPS provides the clearest example of such alternative knowledge communities, both the PGT and DBS cases illuminate similar spaces. Whether these manifest as online forums where prospective parents ask questions and read about others' experiences or in-person support groups where DBS users share practical tips for daily living, the proliferation of these spaces points to an insufficiency in medical establishments and an opportunity to build alternative systems.

Medical technology itself plays an ambivalent role in the production and circulation of discourses and practices about disability. The technologies examined in this book are imbued with neoliberal ableism that demands individuals look, behave, and interact in rigid alignment with ableist paradigms, while they also act as valves to release the pressure of those demands. As Kristina Gupta suggests, this ambivalence may in fact be a key characteristic of medical technology in Western culture. "Because of systemic inequality," she writes, "many, if not all, mainstream medical interventions will simultaneously reinforce social inequality and alleviate some individual suffering."[36] Rhetorics of individual agency and independence mobilize discourses around the development and use of these technologies, and yet users' decisions to pursue them are often driven by feelings of guilt, personal responsibility, and limited options. Encounters with medical technologies cannot be considered in isolation, however. These experiences exist at the interface of bodymind and environment, but also at the interfaces of self and community, human and technology, discourse and materiality. Ignoring the complexities that frame the individual experience of medical technologies obfuscates the sociality embedded in technological interventions. Therefore, offering a prescriptive recommendation for the adoption or rejection of a certain medical technology is neither appropriate nor sufficient. How then, do medical technology users escape this double bind?

Escaping the Double Bind

In the preceding chapters, I have sought to understand the construction and enactment of disability, responsibility, and knowledge when choosing and using of medical technologies to identify and intervene on disabled bodyminds. There is a long history of scholarship arguing that people with nonnormative bodyminds face pressures to more closely approximate hegemonic ideals. These pressures can be social, as in the stigmatizing of nonnormative appearance and movement; political, as when access to the rights of citizenship is contingent on proving ability; or material, as when disabled bodyminds are modified to compensate for nonaccommodating infrastructure. A reliance on medicine to correct these misfittings is linked to the production of the ideal neoliberal subject as self-governing and self-sufficient. Self-governance has become a defining feature in twenty-first-century medicine. As Michelle Murphy writes, "Rather than simply compliant and obedient, the good patient, over the course of the late twentieth century, became someone who was educated enough to ensure doctors had negotiated 'informed consent,' and who could be her or his own advocate, as well as someone who regulated her or his own risk and 'lifestyle' for the sake of good health."[37] Disabled bodyminds are thus unruly and unworthy unless and until they seek "appropriate" medical intervention. The proliferation of medical technologies insists on decisions where previously no choices existed. While the neoliberal logic demands self-responsibility, medicalization undermines the authority of nonexperts to have their decisions taken seriously, particularly if their knowledge or values come into conflict with medical authority. In this double bind, one is expected to be responsible but unable to be authoritative. Self-responsibility for body management under neoliberal ableism essentially means giving oneself over to the recommendations and requirements of a medical authority.

And yet the informants whose stories populate these pages found ways to survive and reshape these ableist systems. Arseli Dokumacı points to this world building through her articulation of "activist affordances," discrete actions taken by disabled people that make uninhabitable worlds momentarily habitable through careful choreography. She argues that these acts are "a precursor to accessible futures that will never take a final material form but will nonetheless arise from constant searching, improvisation, and dreaming."[38] While Dokumacı is careful to distinguish these acts from the use of assistive or medical technology, there is a strong resonance between what she describes and the experiences of medical technology users alleviating the pressures of the durable ableism of a neoliberal society. Such actions, much like the adoption or co-option of medical technologies, are necessary in a world in which disabled people are "made to feel out of place and out of time, bereft of an environment in which they can see a semblance of themselves."[39]

A new embodied knowledge politic requires pushing beyond an analysis of individual experience and intervention, and toward a collective understanding of disability. Kristina Gupta writes that perhaps the path to thriving while occupying a marginalized bodymind is through directing "our feminist, queer, antiracist, and crip activist energies . . . [at] the broader sociopolitical structures that ensure that medical interventions are used largely in the service of normalization and working to ensure that all people, regardless of race, gender, sexuality, class, or ability, have access to the basic resources required to flourish."[40] Dan Goodley too writes extensively about the mobilization of disabled people to resist "neoliberal-able citizenship," calling for further action to examine "the politics of dis/ability as the space for challenging and contesting neoliberal discourse that threatens to get under our skin, colonise our minds and shape political resistance."[41] Melinda Hall imagines futures where enhancements, be they "political, social, or technological," depend not on "ableist discourses of risk that fetishize autonomy and choice and visions of happiness that depend on added capabilities" but on "expression[s] of care, care of existing individuals—not on idealized subjects that cannot, and will not, exist."[42]

Users of PGT, DBS, and DIYAPS adopt these technologies as means to displace the pressures of neoliberal ableism, among other reasons. Therefore, taking their narratives seriously allows us to better identify those sites of oppression. This new embodied knowledge politic demands a less autonomous, more collective subject; less rigid, more fluid conceptions of bodily integrity, knowledge, and authority; and a less deterministic relationship with technology. What happens if, armed with that embodied knowledge, we redirect our technological efforts? Can we resituate technological innovation not to correct misfitting bodyminds but to address the causes of neoliberal ableism at their root? To do so, we must first characterize disruptions in hegemonic power and authority to reframe disability and to cultivate and encourage subaltern disabled knowledge systems. Such a call requires reorienting ourselves to disability and expanding our view of what constitutes a good and desirable life. If such a transformation is possible, then, as Margrit Shildrick writes, "anomalous bodies need no longer be a source of anxiety but hold out the promise of productive new becomings."[43] Disabled lives can and must become less medicalized, and technologies applied to disabled bodyminds can be rooted in values other than pathologization. When the lives of disabled people are depathologized, spaces will open for creating alternative imaginaries—and technologies to power those imaginaries—toward inclusive futures.

Acknowledgments

Like most things in my life, this book is the product of collaboration, interdependence, and community. There are too many people who have given me too much for me to possibly do them justice in this brief space. Please know my gratitude is boundless.

I want to first extend my thanks to all of the informants who contributed their perspectives to build the three cases at the heart of this book. Thank you for your trust, your openness, and your willingness to provide feedback at multiple points in this project. This book would quite literally not be possible without you. I hope I have honored your stories.

Thank you to all the intellectual homes I have had over the years, each contributing an integral piece to the scholar and person I have become. I am fortunate that I discovered disability studies at The Ohio State University when I was eighteen. It changed the trajectory of my life. Thanks especially to Amy Shuman for fostering and directing my undergraduate enthusiasm into a career path. Another stroke of luck found me at the Tizard Center at the University of Kent at Canterbury, where I am thankful to have developed rigorous, justice-oriented qualitative research skills under the compassionate and generous eye of Rachel Forrester-Jones. At Arizona State University, where this project was initially conceived as a dissertation, I am thankful to the many people within the School for the Future of Innovation in Society and the School of Social Transformation who modeled intellectual curiosity, humility, and care in all they do. I was beyond fortunate to have Mary Margaret Fonow as a mentor. Her knowledge, generosity, and warmth bolstered me often, and her tireless efforts to create spaces for marginalized scholars and knowledges in academia have changed many lives, including mine. I am grateful to Emma Frow and Heather Ross for their support throughout the development of this project in its original form, and to Katina Michael, who not only supported me as a graduate student but also first introduced me to recipients of deep brain stimulation. Thank you to Erik Johnston and Dana Lewis, who invited me to contribute to the Opening Pathways project, eventually leading to my case study on do-it-yourself artificial pancreas systems. Thank you as well to the NSF Alliance for Person-Centered Accessible Technologies IGERT team for financial and scholarly support, and especially to Jay Klein, whose influence mattered immensely when I felt adrift during my first semester as a PhD student. Thank you for providing a template for how disability justice can fit into technological spaces.

To colleagues and friends across disability studies, science and technology studies, and gender studies spaces—especially those in the Society for the Social Studies of Science and the Disability Studies Interest Group at the National Women Studies Association—thank you for teaching me, for mentoring me, for challenging me, and for collaborating with me. You are too many to name, but I hope you see your influence in this work.

Since coming to the University of Toledo's Disability Studies Program in 2020, I have pinched myself daily at my good fortune. To contribute to a program composed of brilliant colleagues, passionate students, and deep connections to disabled communities in Northwest Ohio and across the world has been a dream. Thank you to my colleagues Kim Nielsen, Ally Day, Jim Ferris, and Linda Curtis for creating the absolute best department a junior scholar could hope to walk into. Thank you to all my students for making this work so profoundly rewarding—especially the students in my Disability, Technology, and Society course, who endured listening to me talk about the contents of this book for several years. Thinking in community with you all is a gift that I can never repay.

Thank you to everyone at the University of Minnesota Press who made this book possible. A special thanks to Leah Pennywark for your insight, guidance, and support throughout the publishing process and to Anne Carter, Laura Westlund, Judy Selhorst, Carla Valadez, and the many others who helped usher this book through production. Thank you also to Annie Hammang, Jenna Vikse, Chad McDonald, Lynn Wasley, Joey Gamble, Ally Day, Kim Nielsen, Tara Corkery, Sarra Burnham, Sam Shimel, Mateo Pimentel, F Njahîra Wangarî, Mark Monteleone, Brigid Bartlett, Natalie Zanin, Mary Margaret Fonow, Heather Ross, Emma Frow, Katina Michael, Ben

Hurlbut, and the three anonymous readers for commenting on various iterations of this work. Your thoughtful remarks strengthened this book immensely. In a moment when peer review in academia is struggling, I cannot express how meaningful it is to have deep, kind, and supportive recommendations. Thank you for reading my work and for caring to make it better.

So many communities held me up through the development of this manuscript. My thanks to all the friends who nourished my soul and challenged me to be the best version of myself. To Detour Company Theatre and the SALUTE Storytellers, for inviting me into the warmest, most welcoming communities I've been honored to be a part of. To the Toledo Lucas County Public Library, the Tempe Public Library, and all the precious public spaces where I spent countless hours writing, editing, and agonizing. To the animal companions who curled up with me on all the chairs, carpets, beds, and couches on which this manuscript was typed, and who forced me out of myself and into nature when I needed it most: Ace, Hambone, Kif, Jack, Jim, Fatface, and even Ghost Cat. To my family, especially my parents, Mark and Peg, for their support and encouragement in all things. To my sister, Maggie, for being the other half of me. And to Neils, whose love, encouragement, and endless good humor enabled both this book and every other wonderful thing in our shared life.

Notes

INTRODUCTION

1. "Medical technology" is a catchall term that encompasses many kinds of equipment, processes, and laboratory procedures implemented in health care systems—anything from syringes to MRI machines. It is typically used to refer to equipment, processes, or procedures that are employed or implanted in clinics and hospitals, as opposed to assistive or everyday technologies, which are used in other settings.
2. The language regarding disability has historically been a fraught subject, both in theory and in practice. See, for example, Irving Zola, "Self, Identity, and the Naming Question: Reflections on the Language of Disability," *Social Science & Medicine* 36, no. 2 (1993): 167–73. While in the past these controversies have involved the appropriation and degradation of medical terms (for example, "moron" and "feebleminded") and the reclamation of these terms by disabled communities (see the reclamation of "crip" specifically), contemporary debate often centers on the use of person-first language (that is, "person with a disability") versus identity-first language ("disabled person"). Proponents of person-first language, who often include disability service providers, governmental agencies, and medical professionals, argue that it reduces stigma by focusing on the humanity of people with disabilities. For example, the American Psychological Association previously recommended person-first language as a "constructive way to counter negative or ambivalent attitudes toward people with disabilities, shifting them in positive directions, toward openness and understanding," as cited in Dana Dunn and Erin Andrews, "Person-First and Identity-First Language: Developing Psychologists' Cultural Competence Using Disability Language," *American Psychologist* 70, no. 3 (2015): 256. Increasingly, however, both disability theorists and advocacy organizations endorse identity-first language, arguing that person-first language constructs disability as "something you would want separated from you, like a rotten tooth that needs to be pulled out." Cara Liebowitz, "I Am Disabled: On Identity-First vs. Person-First Language," The Body Is Not an Apology, March 20, 2015,

para. 4, https://thebodyisnotanapology.com. Following the convention of both critical disability studies and disabled activists, I use identity-first language when writing about disability in the abstract or as a general term. In instances where I am discussing the specifics of an interview or case, I use the preferred language of the person in question, where it is known.

"Bodymind" is a term increasingly favored in critical disability studies to recognize the inseparability of the mind from the body and to resist the Cartesian dualism that privileges one over the other through the mere act of distinguishing them. Further, the term signifies cognitive and mental difference as a significant unit of analysis, forcing scholars—largely feminist disability studies scholars—to confront the social, political, and ontological implications of "able-mindedness" alongside able-bodiedness. For further discussion, see Margaret Price, "The Bodymind Problem and the Possibilities of Pain," *Hypatia: A Journal of Feminist Philosophy* 30, no. 1 (2015): 268–84.

3. Aimi Hamraie and Kelly Fritsch, "Crip Technoscience Manifesto," *Catalyst: Feminism, Theory, Technoscience* 5, no. 1 (2019), https://catalystjournal.org; Susan Wendell, "Toward a Feminist Theory of Disability," *Hypatia: A Journal of Feminist Philosophy* 4, no. 2 (1989): 104–24; Michael Oliver, "Changing the Social Relations of Research Production?," *Disability, Handicap and Society* 7, no. 2 (1992): 101–14; Rebecca Monteleone, "Beyond Participation: Empowering People with Disabilities in Research and Design," *Technology and Innovation* 20, no. 1 (2018): 133–39.
4. Nicholas D. Jewson, "The Disappearance of the Sick-Man from Medical Cosmology, 1770–1870," *Sociology* 10, no. 2 (1976): 225–44.
5. Adele E. Clarke, Janet K. Shim, Laura Mamo, Jennifer Ruth Fosket, and Jennifer R. Fishman, "Biomedicalization: Technoscientific Transformations of Health, Illness, and U.S. Biomedicine," in *Biomedicalization: Technoscience, Health, and Illness in the U.S.*, ed. Adele E. Clarke, Laura Mamo, Jennifer Ruth Fosket, Jennifer R. Fishman, and Janet K. Shim (Durham, N.C.: Duke University Press, 2010), 47–87.
6. Rebecca Monteleone and Ally Day, "Wearing Danger: Surveillance, Control, and Quantified Healthism in American Medicine," in *FemTech: Intersectional Interventions in Women's Digital Health*, ed. Lindsay Balfour (London: Palgrave Macmillan, 2023), 248.
7. I opt for "technologied" rather than "technologized" here and throughout the book in order to draw attention to the haphazard proliferation of technologies in clinical medicine, as opposed to the intentional process of epistemological and ontological transformation suggested by "technologization."
8. Marika H. F. Burda, Marjan van den Akker, Frans van der Horst, Paul Lemmens, and J. André Knottnerus, "Collecting and Validating

Experiential Expertise Is Doable but Poses Methodological Challenges," *Journal of Clinical Epidemiology* 72 (April 2016): 10–15.

9. Ilana Löwy, *Imperfect Pregnancies: A History of Birth Defects and Prenatal Diagnosis* (Baltimore: Johns Hopkins University Press, 2017), 42.
10. "Prenatal Genetic Diagnostic Tests: FAQs," American College of Obstetricians and Gynecologists, updated December 2022, https://www.acog.org.
11. Löwy, *Imperfect Pregnancies*, 102.
12. "Prenatal Genetic Screening Tests: FAQs," American College of Obstetricians and Gynecologists, updated October 2020, https://www.acog.org; "Carrier Screening: FAQs," American College of Obstetricians and Gynecologists, updated December 2020, https://www.acog.org.
13. Gareth M. Thomas, Barbara Katz Rothman, Heather Strange, and Joanna E. Latimer, "Testing Times: The Social Life of Non-Invasive Prenatal Testing," *Science, Technology and Society* 26, no. 1 (2021): 81–97.
14. "Ob-Gyns Release Revised Recommendations on Screening and Testing for Genetic Disorders," press release, American College of Obstetricians and Gynecologists, March 1, 2016, https://www.acog.org.
15. Megan Raymond, Julie Barbera, Sarah Boudova, Kavita Vinekar, Rebecca Horgan, Rodney McLaren, and Huda Kouatly, "Implications for Prenatal Genetic Testing in the United States after the Reversal of *Roe v. Wade*," *Obstetrics and Gynecology* 141, no. 3 (2023): 445–54.
16. While I focus on genetic counseling in prenatal and preconception settings, genetic counselors operate in many different fields, including pediatrics, oncology, and psychiatry, as well as in research and other nonclinical settings.
17. Daniel Navon, "Genetic Counseling, Activism and 'Genotype-First' Diagnosis of Developmental Disorders," *Journal of Genetic Counseling* 21, no. 6 (2012): 775.
18. Diane Paul, *The Politics of Heredity: Essays on Eugenics, Medicine, and the Nature–Nurture Debate* (Albany: University of New York Press, 1998), 133–56.
19. Paul, *Politics of Heredity*, 148, quoting the Institute of Medicine Committee on Assessing Genetic Risk, "Assessing Genetic Risks: Implications for Health and Social Policy," in *National Academies Collection: Reports Funded by the National Institutes of Health* (Washington, D.C.: National Academies Press, 1994), 14–15.
20. Gareth M. Thomas, *Down's Syndrome Screening and Reproductive Politics: Care, Choice, and Disability in the Prenatal Clinic* (London: Routledge, 2017).
21. See, for example, Carine Vassy, "From a Genetic Innovation to Mass Health Programmes: The Diffusion of Down's Syndrome Prenatal Screening and Diagnostic Techniques in France," *Social Science & Medicine* 63, no. 8 (2006): 2041–51.

22. Rayna Rapp, *Testing Women, Testing the Fetus: The Social Impact of Amniocentesis in America* (New York: Routledge, 1999); Jackie Leach Scully, "Disability and Genetics in the Era of Genomic Medicine," *Nature Reviews Genetics* 9, no. 10 (2008): 797–802.
23. Sandy Sufian and Rosemarie Garland-Thomson, "The Dark Side of CRISPR," *Scientific American,* February 16, 2021, para. 18, https://www.scientificamerican.com.
24. Marsha Saxton, "Disability Rights and Selective Abortion," in *The Disability Studies Reader,* 4th ed., ed. Lennard J. Davis (New York: Routledge, 2013), 87–99.
25. Miguel A. Faria, "Neolithic Trepanation Decoded—A Unifying Hypothesis: Has the Mystery as to Why Primitive Surgeons Performed Cranial Surgery Been Solved?" *Surgical Neurology International* 6, no. 1 (2015): 72. The Neolithic period began around 10,000 BCE and lasted approximately six thousand years.
26. Samir S. Amr and Abdelghani Tbakhi, "Abu Al Qasim Al Zahrawi (Albucasis): Pioneer of Modern Surgery," *Annals of Saudi Medicine* 27, no. 3 (2007): 220–21; Alexandrina Nikova and Theodossios Birbilis, "The Basic Steps of Evolution of Brain Surgery," *Maedica: A Journal of Clinical Medicine* 12, no. 4 (2017): 297–305.
27. Nikova and Birbilis, "Basic Steps of Evolution of Brain Surgery."
28. Modern stereotactic surgery can be completed using frameless stereotactic navigation devices, although stereotactic frames are still commonly used for DBS, as reported by Carla Piano, Francesco Bove, Delia Mulas, Anna Rita Bentivoglio, Beatrice Cioni, and Tommaso Tufo, "Frameless Stereotaxy in Subthalamic Deep Brain Stimulation: 3-Year Clinical Outcome," *Neurological Sciences* 42, no. 1 (2020): 259–66.
29. John Gardner, "A History of Deep Brain Stimulation: Technological Innovation and the Role of Clinical Assessment Tools," *Social Studies of Science* 43, no. 5 (2013): 707–28; Lady Diana Ladino, Syed Rizvi, and José Francisco Téllez-Zenteno, "The Montreal Procedure: The Legacy of the Great Wilder Penfield," *Epilepsy & Behavior* 83 (June 2018): 151–61. Ablation is the intentional destruction of tissue.
30. "Parkinson's Disease," National Institute of Neurological Disorders and Stroke, last reviewed November 28, 2023, https://www.ninds.nih.gov.
31. Maryam Rahman, Gregory J. Murad, and J. Mocco, "Early History of the Stereotactic Apparatus in Neurosurgery," *Neurosurgical Focus* 27, no. 3 (2009): E12.
32. Gardner, "History of Deep Brain Stimulation."
33. Blair Ford, "Deep Brain Stimulation," in *Encyclopedia of Movement Disorders,* ed. Katie Kompoliti and Leonard Verhagen (Cambridge, Mass.: Academic Press, 2010).
34. "Brain Stimulation Therapies for Epilepsy," National Institute of Neu-

rological Disorders and Stroke, February 2023, https://www.ninds.nih.gov; "Humanitarian Device Exemption (HDE): Medtronic (Activa) Deep Brain Stimulation for OCD Therapy," U.S. Food and Drug Administration, February 2009, https://www.accessdata.fda.gov.

35. Ford, "Deep Brain Stimulation"; Hye Ran Park, In Hyang Kim, Hyejin Kang, Dong Soo Lee, Bung-Nyun Kim, Dong Gyu Kim, and Sun Ha Paek, "Nucleus Accumbens Deep Brain Stimulation for a Patient with Self-Injurious Behavior and Autism Spectrum Disorder: Functional and Structural Changes of the Brain; Report of a Case and Review of Literature," *Acta Neurochirurgica* 159, no. 1 (2017): 137–43.
36. Ryszard M. Pluta, Gabriela D. Perazza, and Robert M. Golub, "JAMA Patient Page: Deep Brain Stimulation," *JAMA* 305, no. 7 (2011): 732.
37. Julie G. Pilitis, Olga Khazen, and Shrey Patel, "Deep Brain Stimulation," American Association of Neurological Surgeons, April 15, 2024, https://www.aans.org.
38. "Christine Coles' Patient Story," American Association of Neurological Surgeons, April 30, 2024, para. 2, https://www.aans.org.
39. Anna R. Gagliardi, Pascale Lehoux, Ariel Ducey, Anthony Easty, Sue Ross, Chaim M. Bell, Patricia Trbovich, Julie Takata, and David R. Urbach, "Factors Constraining Patient Engagement in Implantable Medical Device Discussions and Decisions: Interviews with Physicians," *International Journal for Quality in Health Care* 29, no. 2 (2017): 276–82.
40. Frederic Gilbert, Eliza Goddard, John Noel M. Viaña, Adrian Carter, and Malcolm Horne, "I Miss Being Me: Phenomenological Effects of Deep Brain Stimulation," *AJOB Neuroscience* 8, no. 2 (2017): 96–109.
41. John Gardner and Narelle Warren, "Learning from Deep Brain Stimulation: The Fallacy of Techno-Solutionism and the Need for 'Regimes of Care,'" *Medicine, Health Care and Philosophy* 22, no. 3 (2019): 367.
42. Gardner, "History of Deep Brain Stimulation," 709.
43. Marianna Karamanou, Athanase Protogerou, Gregory Tsoucalas, George Androutsos, and Effie Poulakou-Rebelakou, "Milestones in the History of Diabetes Mellitus: The Main Contributors," *World Journal of Diabetes* 10, no. 7 (2016): 1–7.
44. Karamanou et al., "Milestones in the History of Diabetes Mellitus."
45. Linda Bryder and Courtney Harper, "Commentary: More Than 'Tentative Opinions': Harry Himsworth and Defining Diabetes," *International Journal of Epidemiology* 42, no. 6 (2013): 1599–1600.
46. David C. W. Lau, "Diabetes Technology and Devices Transform the Lives of People with Diabetes," *Canadian Journal of Diabetes* 39, no. 3 (2015): 174–75.
47. Klemen Dovc and Tadej Battelino, "Evolution of Diabetes Technology," *Endocrinology and Metabolism Clinics of North America* 49, no. 1 (2019): 1–18.

48. Nicole C. Foster, Roy W. Beck, Kellee M. Miller, Mark A. Clements, Michael R. Rickels, Linda A. DiMeglio, David M. Maahs, William V. Taborlane, Richard Bergenstal, Elizabeth Smith, Beth A. Olson, and Satish K. Garg, "State of Type 1 Diabetes Management and Outcomes from the T1D Exchange in 2016–2018," *Diabetes Technology and Therapeutics* 21, no. 2 (2019): 66–72. The T1D Exchange is a U.S.-based nonprofit that operates a longitudinal research study in which information is collected from Americans with type 1 diabetes through an annual survey.
49. Dovc and Battelino, "Evolution of Diabetes Technology."
50. Guillermo E. Umpierrez and David C. Klonoff, "Diabetes Technology Update: Use of Insulin Pumps and Continuous Glucose Monitoring in the Hospital," *Diabetes Care* 41, no. 8 (2018): 1579–89.
51. Thomas S. J. Crabtree, Alasdair McLay, and Emma G. Wilmot, "DIY Artificial Pancreas Systems: Here to Stay?," *Practical Diabetes* 36, no. 2 (2019): 63–68.
52. While there are differences among the users of OpenAPS, Loop, and AndroidAPS, I consider all users to be part of the overarching DIYAPS community.
53. Crabtree et al., "DIY Artificial Pancreas Systems."
54. Most often, OpenAPS accesses these trends through another open-source program called Autotune, which iteratively adjusts basals, ISF, and carb ratios by drawing on data over several weeks. Dana Lewis, "Autotune (Automatically Assessing Basal Rates, ISF, and Carb Ratio with #OpenAPS—and Even without It!)," DIYPS, January 20, 2017, https://diyps.org.
55. Paul Heltzel, "The Diabetes Patients Who Hacked a Pancreas," *Experience Magazine,* November 13, 2019, https://expmag.com.
56. Dana Lewis, "Open Artificial Pancreas System," TEDxFHKufstein, YouTube, April 11, 2018, https://www.youtube.com.
57. Lewis, "Open Artificial Pancreas System."
58. Jozef Keulartz and Henk van den Belt, "DIY-Bio—Economic, Epistemological and Ethical Implications and Ambivalences," *Life Sciences, Society and Policy* 12 (2016): art. 7.
59. Phil Brown, Stephen Zavestoski, Sabrina McCormick, Brian Mayer, Rachel Morello-Frosch, and Rebecca Gasior Altman, "Embodied Health Movements: New Approaches to Social Movements in Health," *Sociology of Health and Illness* 26, no. 1 (2004): 50–80.
60. Christopher M. Kelty, "Outlaw, Hackers, Victorian Amateurs: Diagnosing Public Participation in the Life Sciences Today," *Journal of Science Communication* 9, no. 1 (2010): 5.
61. Dana Lewis, Scott Leibrand, and #OpenAPS Community, "Real-World Use of Open Source Artificial Pancreas Systems," *Journal of Diabetes Science and Technology* 10, no. 6 (2016): 1411.

62. The term "epistemic injustice" originated with philosopher Miranda Fricker, *Epistemic Injustice: Power and Ethics of Knowing* (Oxford: Oxford University Press, 2007).
63. The interviews were conducted from July 2017 through September 2019. I interviewed thirteen informants in the PGT case, twelve in the DBS case, and sixteen in the DIYAPS case. Samples were intentionally small to allow for the deep analysis favored in inductive qualitative inquiry. A sample size for each case was not determined before data collection began; rather, informant recruitment was ceased on the basis of what Yvonna Lincoln and Egon Guba refer to as "informational redundancy," that point at which no new information relating to the research questions is gained from new interviews. See Yvonna Lincoln and Egon Guba, *Naturalistic Inquiry* (Newbury Park, Calif.: SAGE, 1985). I recruited informants through online and in-person support, patient, and professional organizations; responses to physical flyers; and my existing professional network. Additional informants were recruited through snowball sampling when suggestions were made spontaneously during the interview process. Several of the informants were previously known to me, though none in professional relationships that would contribute to a conflict of interest.
64. In the case of PGT, the secondary informants were prenatal genetic counselors. In the case of DBS, they included several spouses who were also acting as caregivers. In the case of DIYAPS, several informants were parents who built and used DIY tech for their minor children. Additionally, some of the DIYAPS users were also working professionally in diabetes technology development as designers, engineers, or researchers.
65. I provide a summary of the types of documents evaluated in the endnotes for each case study chapter.
66. Jack Halberstam, *Female Masculinity* (Durham, N.C.: Duke University Press, 1998), 13.
67. Barney G. Glaser and Anselm L. Strauss, *The Discovery of Grounded Theory: Strategies for Qualitative Research* (New Brunswick, N.J.: Aldine, 1967).
68. Andrea Vick, "The Embodied Experience of Episodic Disability among Women with Multiple Sclerosis," *Disability and Society* 28, no. 2 (2013): 176–89.
69. Jae Hoon Lim, "Qualitative Methods in Adult Development and Learning: Theoretical Traditions, Current Practices, and Emerging Horizons," in *The Oxford Handbook of Reciprocal Adult Development and Learning*, 2nd ed., ed. Carol Hoare (Oxford: Oxford University Press, 2011), 40–60.
70. Renate M. Kahlke, "Generic Qualitative Approaches: Pitfalls and

Benefits of Methodological Mixology," *International Journal of Qualitative Methods* 13, no. 1 (2014): 47.
71. Caroline Ramazanoglu and Janet Holland, "Tripping over Experience: Some Problems in Feminist Epistemology," *Discourse: Studies in the Cultural Politics of Education* 20, no. 3 (1999): 381–92.
72. Banu Subramaniam, Laura Foster, Sandra Harding, Deboleena Roy, and Kim TallBear, "Feminism, Postcolonialism, Technoscience," in *The Handbook of Science and Technology Studies,* 4th ed., ed. Ulrike Felt, Rayvon Fouché, Clark A. Miller, and Laurel Smith-Doerr (Cambridge: MIT Press, 2017), 407–33.
73. Prenatal genetic counselors were interviewed under a different protocol and received the final draft but not their transcripts. Approximately 70 percent of informants who received their transcripts requested edits, all of which were accepted. Approximately 20 percent of informants provided feedback on the early draft of this monograph. Their comments have informed the final version, particularly in chapters 3, 4, and 5.
74. Linda Birt, Suzanne Scott, Debbie Cavers, Christine Campbell, and Fiona Walter, "Member Checking: A Tool to Enhance Trustworthiness or Merely a Nod to Validation," *Qualitative Health Research* 26, no. 13 (2016): 1802–11.

1. THE ACCEPTABLE BODYMIND IN A TECHNOLOGIED WORLD

1. Simi Linton, *Claiming Disability: Knowledge and Identity* (New York: New York University Press, 1998), 2.
2. Wendell, "Toward a Feminist Theory of Disability," 110.
3. Erving Goffman, *Frame Analysis: An Essay on the Organization of Experience* (Cambridge, Mass.: Harvard University Press, 1974).
4. Goffman, *Frame Analysis,* 39.
5. Marno Retief and Rantoa Letšosa, "Models of Disability: A Brief Overview," *HTS Teologiese Studies / Theological Studies* 74, no. 1 (2018): E1–E8.
6. Monteleone and Day, "Wearing Danger," 237–55.
7. Peter Conrad, "Medicalization and Social Control," *Annual Review of Sociology* 18, no. 1 (1992): 209–32.
8. Leo Marx, "Does Improved Technology Mean Progress?," *Technology Review,* January 1987, 33–41.
9. Eric Shyman, "The Reinforcement of Ableism: Normality, the Medical Model of Disability, and Humanism in Applied Behavior Analysis and ASD," *Intellectual and Developmental Disabilities* 54, no. 5 (2016): 366–76.
10. Wendell, "Toward a Feminist Theory of Disability," 110.
11. Alison Kafer, *Feminist, Queer, Crip* (Bloomington: Indiana University Press, 2013), 27.

12. Rapp, *Testing Women.*
13. Union of the Physically Impaired Against Segregation and the Disability Alliance, *Fundamental Principles of Disability* (London, 1975), 3, available at Centre for Disability Studies, University of Leeds, https://disability-studies.leeds.ac.uk.
14. Tom Shakespeare, "The Social Model of Disability," in *The Disability Studies Reader,* 3rd ed., ed. Lennard J. Davis (New York: Routledge, 2010), 216.
15. Shakespeare, "Social Model of Disability," 218.
16. Moya Bailey and Izetta Autumn Mobley, "Work in the Intersections: A Black Feminist Disability Framework," *Gender & Society* 33, no. 2 (2019): 28.
17. Tobin Siebers, "Disability and the Theory of Complex Embodiment: For Identity Politics in a New Register," in Davis, *Disability Studies Reader,* 3rd ed., 284.
18. Kafer, *Feminist, Queer, Crip,* 9.
19. Siebers, "Disability and the Theory of Complex Embodiment," 273.
20. Gregor Wolbring, "Ableism," in *Encyclopedia of Nanoscience and Society,* ed. David H. Guston (Thousand Oaks, Calif.: SAGE, 2010), 2.
21. Michael Bratton, "Neoliberalism," in *International Encyclopedia of Political Science,* ed. Bertrand Badie, Dirk Berg-Schlosser, and Leonardo Morlino (Thousand Oaks, Calif.: SAGE, 2011), 1676.
22. Dan Goodley, *Dis/Ability Studies: Theorising Disablism and Ableism* (London: Routledge, 2014), 26.
23. Goodley, *Dis/Ability Studies,* 63.
24. Goodley, *Dis/Ability Studies,* 23.
25. Merri Lisa Johnson and Robert McRuer, "Cripistemologies: Introduction," *Journal of Literary and Cultural Disability Studies* 8, no. 2 (2014): 137.
26. Richard Devlin and Dianne Pothier, "Introduction: Toward a Critical Theory of Dis-Citizenship," in *Critical Disability Theory: Essays in Philosophy, Politics, Policy, and Law,* ed. Dianne Pothier and Richard Devlin (Vancouver: UBC Press, 2006), 1.
27. Devlin and Pothier, "Introduction," 18.
28. Bailey and Mobley, "Work in the Intersections," 7.
29. Kristin Bumiller, "The Geneticization of Autism: From New Reproductive Technologies to the Conception of Genetic Normalcy," *Signs:* Journal of Women in Culture and Society 34, no. 4 (2009): 290.
30. Ann Kerr and Tom Shakespeare, *Genetic Politics: From Eugenics to Genome* (Cheltenham: New Clarion Press, 2002), 136.
31. Melinda Hall, *The Bioethics of Enhancement: Transhumanism, Disability, and Biopolitics* (Lanham, Md.: Lexington Books, 2016), 66.
32. Kerr and Shakespeare, *Genetic Politics,* 100.
33. For more on this, see Goodley, *Dis/Ability Studies.*
34. Michelle Murphy, *Seizing the Means of Reproduction: Entanglements of*

Feminism, Health, and Technoscience (Durham, N.C.: Duke University Press, 2012), 118.

35. On the confusion of technological progress with social good, see Merritt Roe Smith, "Technological Determinism in American Culture," in *Does Technology Drive History? The Dilemma of Technological Determinism,* ed. Merritt Roe Smith and Leo Marx (Cambridge: MIT Press, 1994), 1–35.
36. Peter Conrad, *The Medicalization of Society: On the Transformation of Human Conditions into Treatable Conditions* (Baltimore: Johns Hopkins University Press, 2007), 6.
37. James G. Carrier, "Masking the Social in Educational Knowledge: The Case of Learning Disability Theory," *American Journal of Sociology* 88, no. 5 (1983): 952.
38. Scully, "Disability and Genetics."
39. Peter Conrad and Joseph W. Schneider, *Deviance and Medicalization: From Badness to Sickness* (Philadelphia: Temple University Press, 1992), 8.
40. Susan Wendell, *The Rejected Body: Feminist Philosophical Reflections on Disability* (New York: Routledge, 1996).
41. Grace Hong, *Death beyond Disavowal: The Impossible Politics of Difference* (Minneapolis: University of Minnesota Press, 2015).
42. Gregory Bowker and Susan Leigh Star, *Sorting Things Out: Classification and Its Consequences* (Cambridge: MIT Press, 1999), 210, quoting Muriel Horrell, *Race Classification in South Africa: Its Effects on Human Beings, No.* 2 (Johannesburg: South African Institute of Race Relations, 1958), 77.
43. Wendell, "Toward a Feminist Theory of Disability."
44. Bowker and Star, *Sorting Things Out,* 5.
45. Kristina Gupta, *Medical Entanglements: Rethinking Feminist Debates about Healthcare* (New Brunswick, N.J.: Rutgers University Press, 2020), 25.
46. Clarke et al., "Biomedicalization," 47.
47. Conrad, "Medicalization and Social Control"; Carrier, "Masking the Social in Educational Knowledge."
48. Mariachiara Tallacchini, "Risk and Rights in Xenotransplantation," in *Reframing Rights: Bioconstitutionalism in the Genetic Age,* ed. Sheila Jasanoff (Cambridge: MIT Press, 2011), 170. Xenotransplantation is the transplantation to a human of tissue from a nonhuman animal source, such as a pig, or of human tissue grown using a nonhuman animal source.
49. Angela Willey, Banu Subramaniam, Jennifer Hamilton, and Jane Couperus, "The Mating Life of Geeks: Love, Neuroscience, and the New Autistic Subject," *Signs: Journal of Women in Culture and Society* 40, no. 2 (2015): 369–91.

50. Tiago Moreira and Paolo Palladino, "Between Truth and Hope: On Parkinson's Disease, Neurotransplantation, and the Production of the 'Self,'" *History of the Human Sciences* 18, no. 3 (2005): 57.
51. John Gardner, Gabrielle Samuel, and Clare Williams, "Sociology of Low Expectations: Recalibration as Innovation Work in Biomedicine," *Science, Technology, & Human Values* 40, no. 6 (2015): 1016.
52. Clarke et al., "Biomedicalization," 51.
53. Langdon Winner, *The Whale and the Reactor: In Search of Limits in an Age of High Technology* (Chicago: University of Chicago Press, 1984), 19–39.
54. Ashley Shew, "Ableism, Technoableism, and Future AI," *IEEE Technology and Society Magazine* 39, no. 1 (2020): 45–46.
55. Clarke et al., "Biomedicalization."
56. Gardner, "History of Deep Brain Stimulation," 723.
57. Robert A. Aronowitz, "The Converged Experience of Risk and Disease," *Milbank Quarterly* 87, no. 2 (2009): 417–42.
58. Robert A. Aronowitz, "When Do Symptoms Become a Disease?," *Annals of Internal Medicine* 9, no. 2 (2001): 803–8.
59. Trevor J. Pinch and Wiebe E. Bijker, "The Social Construction of Facts and Artefacts: Or How the Sociology of Science and the Sociology of Technology Might Benefit Each Other," *Social Studies of Science* 14, no. 3 (1984): 428.
60. Löwy, *Imperfect Pregnancies,* 186.
61. Bruno Latour, *We Have Never Been Modern* (Cambridge, Mass.: Harvard University Press, 1993), 1–12.
62. Karen Barad, "Posthumanist Performativity: Toward an Understanding of How Matter Comes to Matter," *Signs: Journal of Women in Culture and Society* 28, no. 3 (2003): 822.
63. Barad, "Posthumanist Performativity," 808.
64. Sandra Harding, *Whose Science / Whose Knowledge?* (Milton Keynes: Open University Press, 1991), 1–16.
65. Donna Haraway, "Situated Knowledges: The Science Question in Feminism and the Privilege of Partial Perspective," *Feminist Studies* 14, no. 3 (1988): 575–99.
66. Sandra Harding, "'Strong Objectivity': A Response to the New Objectivity Question," *Synthese* 104, no. 3 (1995): 335.
67. Harding, "'Strong Objectivity,'" 341.
68. For more feminist discussion of positionality and knowledge production, see Patricia Hill Collins, "Learning from the Outsider Within: The Sociological Significance of Black Feminist Thought," *Social Problems* 33, no. 6 (1986): S14–S32; Dorothy Smith, *The Everyday World as Problematic: A Feminist Sociology* (Boston: Northeastern University Press, 1987); Haraway, "Situated Knowledges."
69. Pinch and Bijker, "Social Construction of Facts and Artefacts," 19.

70. Bowker and Star, *Sorting Things Out,* 289.
71. Rosemarie Garland-Thomson, "Misfits: A Feminist Materialist Disability Concept," *Hypatia: A Journal of Feminist Philosophy* 26, no. 3 (2011): 594.
72. Siebers, "Disability and the Theory of Complex Embodiment," 273, 278.

2. BECOMING RESPONSIBLE WITH PRENATAL GENETIC TESTING

1. I interviewed thirteen informants for this case, including five users (prospective or current parents), seven practicing genetic counselors, and one medical genetic researcher specializing in prenatal genetic testing, screening, and therapy. Of the five users, four identified as female and one identified as male; three were pregnant at the time of their interviews. Users were recruited through convenience sampling among members of my own personal and professional network, which is reflected in their demographics: while geographically diverse, they were all middle- to upper-middle-class, with higher education and stable employment. The majority were working in higher education at the time of their interviews. I discuss this limitation, and the specific role PGT plays among people in this demographic, at the end of the chapter. One interviewee had never been pregnant and instead shared her experiences with preimplantation and carrier screening during fertility treatments. Of the professionals, seven identified as female and one identified as male. All identified as white. Four of the interviews were conducted in person and the remainder were conducted via videoconferencing or phone call. Interviews with users ranged from forty-five minutes to two hours, averaging seventy minutes. Interviews with professionals ranged from thirty to ninety minutes, averaging approximately one hour. Each of the interviews was conducted in a single session. Quotations from informants in this chapter include comments that some of them made after receiving an early draft of the chapter.

   I also analyzed approximately 204 pages of documentation (forty-one individual documents) from fourteen different sources, including genetic counseling professional organizations, commercial genetic testing companies, hospitals and health care systems, and a government agency. The documents ranged in length from a single page to thirty-eight pages and were of many different types: descriptions of various procedures/technologies, user guidance and recommendations, FAQ pages, user stories, fact sheets, and blogs. I included one set of documents from a commercial company directed at clinicians rather than users because it was publicly available on the same web page as user-directed documents, and so it is reasonable to assume that users can and do access it.

2. Megan Allyse, Mollie A. Minear, Elisa Berson, Shilpa Sridhar, Margaret Rote, Anthony Hung, and Subhashini Chandrasekharan, "Non-Invasive Prenatal Testing: A Review of International Implementation and Challenges," *International Journal of Women's Health* 7 (2015): 113–26.
3. "FDA Warns of Risks Associated with Non-Invasive Prenatal Screening Tests," press release, U.S. Food and Drug Administration, April 19, 2022, https://www.fda.gov.
4. Catherine Joynson, "Our Concerns about Non-Invasive Prenatal Testing (NIPT) in the Private Healthcare Sector," Nuffield Council on Bioethics, February 8, 2019, https://www.nuffieldbioethics.org.
5. Megan Molteni, "How Much Prenatal Genetic Information Do You Actually Want?," *Wired,* March 27, 2019, https://www.wired.com.
6. "Amniocentesis," Mayo Clinic, October 7, 2022, https://www.mayoclinic.org.
7. No genetic counselor in this study disclosed having a disability.
8. Stella Young, "We're Not Here for Your Inspiration," *ABC News,* July 3, 2012, https://www.abc.net.au.
9. Thomas, *Down's Syndrome Screening.*
10. Barbara Katz Rothman, *The Tentative Pregnancy: Prenatal Diagnosis and the Future of Motherhood* (New York: Viking Penguin, 1986).
11. Guido de Wert, Wybo Dondorp, and Diana W. Bianchi, "Fetal Therapy for Down Syndrome: An Ethical Exploration," *Prenatal Diagnosis* 37, no. 3 (2017): 222–28.
12. Saxton, "Disability Rights and Selective Abortion," 95.
13. See, for example, Rapp, *Testing Women*; Alexandra Minna Stern, *Eugenic Nation: Faults and Frontiers of Better Breeding in Modern America* (Berkeley: University of California Press, 2005); Laura Briggs, *How All Politics Became Reproductive Politics: From Welfare Reform to Foreclosure to Trump* (Berkeley: University of California Press, 2017).
14. Nearly all prospective parents in this case had attained some sort of postsecondary or graduate degree and/or were working in higher education settings.
15. For an in-depth discussion of delayed pregnancy and class, see Briggs, *How All Politics Became Reproductive Politics,* 101–48.
16. Kafer, *Feminist, Queer, Crip,* 69.
17. Regrettably, I cannot attend deeply to the racialized dimensions of pregnancy management in this chapter, in part because all of my informants identified as white. As such, both I (as a white researcher) and my informants had the privilege of invisibilizing our racialized experiences. See Peggy McIntosh, "White Privilege: Unpacking the

Invisible Knapsack," *Peace and Freedom Magazine,* July/August, 1989, 10–12. Substantial previous research has examined how the racialized experiences of pregnant people influence the ways in which they understand, interpret, and engage with prenatal testing and screening, as well as their overall experiences of pregnancy and reproductive responsibility. See, for example, Dorothy Wertz, Janet Rosenfield, Sally Janes, and Richard Erbe, "Attitudes toward Abortion among Parents of Children with Cystic Fibrosis," *American Journal of Public Health* 81, no. 8 (1991): 992-996; Carole H. Browner, H. Mabel Preloran, and Simon J. Cox, "Ethnicity, Bioethics, and Prenatal Diagnosis: The Amniocentesis Decisions of Mexican-Origin Women and Their Partners," *American Journal of Public Health* 89, no. 11 (1999): 1658–66; Allison S. Bryant, Mary E. Norton, Sanae Nakagawa, Judith T. Bishop, Sherri Pena, Steven E. Gregorich, and Miriam Kuppermann, "Variation in Women's Understanding of Prenatal Testing," *Obstetrics and Gynecology* 125, no. 6 (2015): 1306–12; Khiara M. Bridges, *Reproducing Race: An Ethnography of Pregnancy as a Site of Racialization* (Berkeley: University of California Press, 2011); Valerie Hartouni, *Cultural Conceptions: On Reproductive Technologies and the Remaking of Life* (Minneapolis: University of Minnesota Press, 1997); Briggs, *How All Politics Became Reproductive Politics.* The absence of the perspectives of people of color is a substantial limitation of this case, and future work is needed in this area. For more on how race becomes embedded in pregnancy and reproductive technologies, see especially Bridges, *Reproducing Race*; Dorothy Roberts, *Killing the Black Body: Race, Reproduction, and the Meaning of Liberty* (New York: Pantheon Books, 1997).

18. Maria Tsouroufli, "Routinisation and Constraints on Informed Choice in a One-Stop Clinic Offering First Trimester Chromosomal Antenatal Screening for Down's Syndrome," *Midwifery* 27, no. 4 (2011): 431–36.
19. Rayna Rapp, "Extra Chromosomes and Blue Tulips: Medico-Familial Interpretations," in *Living and Working with the New Medical Technologies: Intersections of Inquiry,* ed. Margaret Lock, Allen Young, and Alberto Cambrosio (Cambridge: Cambridge University Press, 2009), 184–208; Linn Getz and Anne Luise Kirkengen, "Ultrasound Screening in Pregnancy: Advancing Technology, Soft Markers for Fetal Chromosomal Aberrations, and Unacknowledged Ethical Dilemmas," *Social Science & Medicine* 56, no. 10 (2003): 2045–57; Sarah Franklin, *Embodied Progress: A Cultural Account of Assisted Conception* (London: Routledge, 1997).
20. Annette Patterson and Martha Satz, "Genetic Counseling and the Disabled: Feminism Examines the Stance of Those Who Stand at the Gate," *Hypatia: A Journal of Feminist Philosophy* 17, no. 3 (2002): 123.
21. Edward L. Raab, "The Parameters of Informed Consent," *Transactions of the American Ophthalmological Society* 102 (2004): 225–32.

22. Raab, "Parameters of Informed Consent," 227.
23. Franklin, *Embodied Progress,* 330.
24. Michael Bérubé, "Disability, Democracy, and the New Genetics," in Davis, *Disability Studies Reader,* 3rd ed., 99.
25. Paul, *Politics of Heredity.*
26. Stern, *Eugenic Nation,* 153.
27. Paul, *Politics of Heredity,* 149.
28. Rapp, *Testing Women,* 306. While Rapp refers to "women," I take it for granted that this category includes people of all genders capable of conceiving and carrying a pregnancy.
29. Rapp, *Testing Women,* 318–19.
30. Saxton, "Disability Rights and Selective Abortion," 93.
31. Stern, *Eugenic Nation,* 215.
32. Elizabeth Barnes, *The Minority Body: A Theory of Disability* (Oxford: Oxford University Press, 2016), 139.
33. Jackie Leach Scully, "From 'She Would Say That, Wouldn't She?' to 'Does She Take Sugar?': Epistemic Injustice and Disability," *International Journal of Feminist Approaches to Bioethics* 11, no. 1 (2018): 110.
34. "Genetic Testing of Minors for Adult-Onset Conditions," National Society of Genetic Counselors, April 12, 2018, https://www.nsgc.org.
35. Hall, *Bioethics of Enhancement,* 122.

3. LOSING AND TAKING CONTROL WITH DEEP BRAIN STIMULATION

1. Six of the DBS users identified as male; three identified as female. Three partners identified as female and one as male. All informants were white. Six informants received DBS for Parkinson's disease (George, Fred, Marty, Lynn, Mary, and John), one for torticollis (Carl), one for inherited torsion dystonia (Vickie), and one for chronic pain following a stroke (Bradley). Informants ranged in age from thirty-four (Bradley) to seventy-five (John) and were geographically dispersed across the United States. Informants receiving DBS for reasons other than Parkinson's tended to be younger.

   I examined approximately 187 pages of documentation (seventy-two individual documents) from fifteen sources, which included health systems such as university hospitals and specialized neurological clinics. Documents ranged in length from one to eleven pages. The types of documents encompassed procedure/technology descriptions, user recommendations, fact sheets, patient booklets, user stories, blogs and news stories, research output summaries, FAQs, and a summary of a public event. All were publicly available and searchable.
2. Sosipatros Bratsos, Dimitrios Karponis, and Sohag N. Saleh, "Efficacy and Safety of Deep Brain Stimulation in the Treatment of Parkinson's

Disease: A Systematic Review and Meta-Analysis of Randomized Controlled Trials," *Cureus* 10, no. 10 (2018): 15.

3. Frederick L. Hitti, Ashwin G. Ramayya, Brendan J. McShane, Andrew I. Yang, Kerry A. Vaughan, and Gordon H. Baltuch, "Long-Term Outcomes Following Deep Brain Stimulation for Parkinson's Disease," *Journal of Neurosurgery* 132, no. 1 (2019): 205–10.
4. Frances M. Weaver, Kevin T. Stroupe, Bridget Smith, Beverly Gonzalez, Zhiping Huo, Lishan Cao, Dolores Ippolito, and Kenneth A. Follett, "Survival in Patients with Parkinson's Disease After Deep Brain Stimulation or Medical Management," *Movement Disorders* 32, no. 12 (2017): 1756–63.
5. Jonathan Mathers, Caroline Rick, Crispin Jenkinson, Ruth Garside, Hardev Pall, Rosalind Mitchell, Susan Elizabeth Bayliss, and Laura Jones, "Patients' Experiences of Deep Brain Stimulation for Parkinson's Disease: A Qualitative Systematic Review and Synthesis," *BMJ Open* 6, no. 6 (2016): 1–10.
6. Franziska Maier, Catharine J. Lewis, Nina Horstkoetter, Carsten Eggers, Till A. Dembek, Veerle Visser-Vandewalle, Jens Kuhn, Mateusz Zurowski, Elena Moro, Christiane Woopen, and Lars Timmermann, "Subjective Perceived Outcome of Subthalamic Deep Brain Stimulation in Parkinson's Disease One Year After Surgery," *Parkinsonism & Related Disorders* 24 (2016): 41–47.
7. Malco Rossi, Verónica Bruno, Julieta Arena, Ángel Cammarota, and Marcelo Merello, "Challenges in PD Patient Management After DBS: A Pragmatic Review," *Movement Disorders Clinical Practice* 5, no. 3 (2018): 247.
8. Markus Christen, Merlin Bittlinger, Henrik Walter, Peter Brugger, and Sabine Müller, "Dealing with Side Effects of Deep Brain Stimulation: Lessons Learned from Stimulating the STN," *AJOB Neuroscience* 3, no. 1 (2012): 37.
9. Pilitis et al., "Deep Brain Stimulation."
10. Donatus Cyron, "Mental Side Effects of Deep Brain Stimulation (DBS) for Movement Disorders: The Futility of Denial," *Frontiers in Integrative Neuroscience* 10, no. 17 (2016): 1–4.
11. Cyron, "Mental Side Effects of Deep Brain Stimulation."
12. Rossi et al., "Challenges in PD Patient Management." The sites of implantation vary depending on the precipitating condition, targeted symptoms, and other factors.
13. Brastos et al., "Efficacy and Safety of Deep Brain Stimulation." These authors caution that while adverse events such as infection can be tied directly to the device, in the case of suicide or psychosis, no such clear link exists; such an outcome may be related to the device, or to the disease, to medication, or to external factors.
14. Gilbert et al., "I Miss Being Me."
15. Mathers et al., "Patients' Experiences of Deep Brain Stimulation."

16. Gun-Marie Hariz, Patricia Limousin, and Katarina Hamberg, "'DBS Means Everything—for Some Time': Patients' Perspectives on Daily Life with Deep Brain Stimulation for Parkinson's Disease," *Journal of Parkinson's Disease* 6, no. 2 (2016): 344, citing Gun-Marie Hariz and Lars Forsgren, "Activities of Daily Living and Quality of Life in Persons with Newly Diagnosed Parkinson's Disease According to Subtype of Disease, and in Comparison to Healthy Controls," *Acta Neurologica Scandinavica* 123, no. 1 (2011): 20–27; and S. M. Aquilonius, "Rörelsestörningar," in *Neurologi*, 4th ed., ed. J. Fagius and S. M. Aquilonius (Stockholm: Almqvist & Wiksell, 2006).
17. Daniel Alfonso, Laura Y. Cabrera, Christos Sidiropolous, Fei Wang, and Harini Sarva, "How Parkinson's Patients in the USA Perceive Deep Brain Stimulation in the 21st Century: Results of a Nationwide Survey," *Journal of Clinical Neuroscience* 95 (2022): 20–26.
18. Goodley, *Dis/Ability Studies*, 63.
19. Smith, "Technological Determinism in American Culture"; Clarke et al., "Biomedicalization."
20. Robert McRuer, *Crip Theory: Cultural Signs of Queerness and Disability* (New York: New York University Press, 2006), 88.
21. McRuer, *Crip Theory*, 93.
22. Kafer, *Feminist, Queer, Crip*, 80.
23. Samuel W. Cramer, Truong H. Do, Elise F. Palzer, Anant Naik, Abigail L. Rice, Savannah G. Novy, Jacob T. Hanson, Amber N. Piazza, Madeleine A. Howard, Jared D. Huling, Clark C. Chen, and Robert A. McGovern, "Persistent Racial Disparities in Deep Brain Stimulation for Parkinson's Disease," *Annals of Neurology* 92, no. 2 (2022): 246–54.
24. See Julie-Ann Scott, "Illuminating the Vulnerability of Hegemonic Masculinity through a Performance Analysis of Physically Disabled Men's Personal Narratives," *Disability Studies Quarterly* 34, no. 1 (2014), https://dsq-sds.org.
25. Helen Meekosha, "Gender, International," in *Encyclopedia of Disability*, ed. Gary L. Albrecht (Thousand Oaks, Calif.: SAGE, 2006), 765.
26. R. W. Connell and James W. Messerschmidt, "Hegemonic Masculinity: Rethinking the Concept," *Gender & Society* 19, no. 6 (2005): 829–59.
27. Hariz et al., "'DBS Means Everything.'"
28. Thomas Abrams, "Cartesian Dualism and Disabled Phenomenology," *Scandinavian Journal of Disability Journalism* 18, no. 2 (2016): 118–28.
29. Winner, *The Whale and the Reactor*, 19.

4. REIMAGINING AGENCY WITH DO-IT-YOURSELF ARTIFICIAL PANCREAS SYSTEMS

1. Six users and four guardians identified as female, and four users and two guardians identified as male. Three informants were employed by companies that were commercializing technologies emerging from

DIY spaces. One informant, in addition to being a DIYAPS user, had contributed to research for, about, and by users. Two informants were medical professionals, and two others were in school for medical professions. All but one informant used one of three systems: AndroidAPS, OpenAPS, or Loop. The remaining informant was interviewed immediately prior to beginning use of OpenAPS. Nine informants were living in the United States at the time of their interviews, and the remaining seven were living in Europe. Countries represented were the United Kingdom (two informants), Romania (one), Austria (one), Spain (one), and the Czech Republic (two). Interviews were conducted verbally, in person, over the phone, or via videoconferencing, and ranged from forty to one hundred minutes in length, averaging seventy minutes. In two cases, written correspondence was also included in the data analysis with the informants' permission. One informant requested a follow-up interview, but all other interviews were conducted in single sessions.

I analyzed approximately 262 pages of documentation (twelve individual documents) from six different sources. The majority of materials (224 pages) were user-directed guidance for building and using the three DIY systems. The remaining documents included FAQs, blog posts, press releases, and an official regulatory statement from a U.S. federal agency.

2. Lewis, "Open Artificial Pancreas System"; Dana Lewis, "History and Perspective on DIY Closed Looping," *Journal of Diabetes Science and Technology* 13, no. 4 (2019): 790–93.
3. "OpenAPS Outcomes," OpenAPS, 2024, https://openaps.org.
4. Dana M. Lewis, Richard S. Swain, and Thomas W. Donner, "Improvements in A1C and Time-in-Range in DIY Closed-Loop (OpenAPS) Users," *Diabetes* 67, Supplement 1 (2018): 352-OR. A1C is a measure of the percentage of glycated hemoglobin, blood proteins that are chemically linked to sugars, and "time in range" refers to the number of hours when blood glucose is within the clinically defined range of 70–180 milligrams per deciliter.
5. Vincenzo Provenzano, Edoardo Guastamacchia, Davide Brancato, Gerardo Cappiello, Antonio Maiolo, Raffaele Mancini, Giuseppe Crispino, Ariella De Monte, Salvatore Turco, and Giancarlo Tonolo, "Closing the Loop with OpenAPS in People with Type 1 Diabetes: Experience from Italy," *Diabetes* 67, Supplement 1 (2018): 993-P.
6. Soo Bong Choi, Eun Shil Hong, and Yun Hee Noh, "Open Artificial Pancreas System Reduced Hypoglycemia and Improved Glycemic Control in Patients with Type 1 Diabetes," *Diabetes* 67, Supplement 1 (2018): 964-P.
7. Lewis et al., "Real-World Use," 1411.

8. Lewis et al., "Real-World Use"; Crabtree et al., "DIY Artificial Pancreas Systems."
9. Gregory Goodwin, Gretchen Waldman, Justine Lyons, Adeolu Oladunjoye, and Garry Steil, "OR14-5 Challenges in Implementing Hybrid Closed Loop Insulin Pump Therapy (Medtronic 670g) in a 'Real World' Clinical Setting," *Journal of the Endocrine Society* 3, Supplement 1 (2019): 5.
10. Howard Look, "Tidepool Loop Has Received FDA Clearance!," Tidepool, January 24, 2023, https://www.tidepool.org/blog.
11. Dovc and Battelino, "Evolution of Diabetes Technology."
12. "Blackboxing" refers to the invisibilization of the obfuscation of technological and scientific processes, in part because of their ostensible efficiency. Bruno Latour, *Pandora's Hope: Essays on the Reality of Science Studies* (Cambridge, Mass.: Harvard University Press, 1999), 304.
13. "FDA Warns Against the Use of Unauthorized Devices for Diabetes Management," press release, U.S. Food and Drug Administration, May 17, 2019, https://www.fda.gov.
14. "Medtronic MiniMed 508 and Paradigm Series Insulin Pumps," ICS medical advisory, Cybersecurity and Infrastructure Security Agency, June 27, 2019, https://www.cisa.gov.
15. Melody provided a written response, as the 2019 statement was released after her initial interview.
16. "CE approved" refers to compliance with the protection standards of the European Economic Area, where all goods sold must carry the CE mark. (CE stands for *conformité européenne,* meaning "European conformity.")
17. Keulartz and van den Belt, "DIY-Bio."
18. Annabelle E. Wilcox, Kasia J. Lipska, Stuart K. Weinzimer, Jasmine Gujral, Andrew Arakaki, Linda Kerandi, and Laura M. Nally, "Navigating Barriers to Affording and Obtaining Insulin and Diabetes Supplies," *Journal of Diabetes* 15, no. 1 (2023): 71–75.
19. Allison C. Carey, Pamela Block, and Richard K. Scotch, "Sometimes Allies: Parent-Led Disability Organizations and Social Movements," *Disability Studies Quarterly* 39, no. 1 (2019), https://dsq-sds.org.
20. Regarding vision impairments, a 2015 meta-analysis found that diabetic retinopathy, a leading cause of vision loss, was present in 36 to 94 percent of people with T1D in the United States and Europe, with 7 to 35 percent of people with T1D having their vision affected. Ryan Lee, Tien Y. Wong, and Charumathi Sabanayagam, "Epidemiology of Diabetic Retinopathy, Diabetic Macular Edema and Related Vision Loss," *Eye and Vision* 2, no. 17 (2015): 1–25. In terms of motor skills issues that could have an impact on participation in DIY communities or in building DIYAPS rigs, diabetic cheiroarthropathy (a condition

that can limit a person's ability to flex or extend the fingers) occurs in 8 to 50 percent of people with diabetes (types 1 and 2). Rabia Cherqaoui, Sheldon McKenzie, and Gail Nunlee-Bland, "Diabetic Cheiroarthropathy: A Case Report and Review of the Literature," *Case Reports in Endocrinology* (2013), https://onlinelibrary.wiley.com.

21. Hamraie and Fritsch, "Crip Technoscience Manifesto," 1.
22. Hamraie and Fritsch, "Crip Technoscience Manifesto," 7.
23. M. Remi Yergeau, "Disability Hacktivism," in "Hacking the Classroom: Eight Perspectives," ed. Mary Hocks and Jentery Sayers, *Computers and Composition Online* (2014): para. 27, http://cconlinejournal.org/hacking.
24. Hamraie and Fritsch, "Crip Technoscience Manifesto," 4.
25. Gupta, *Medical Entanglements,* 33.
26. Phil Brown, Rachel Morello-Frosch, Stephen Zavestoski, Sabrina McCormick, Brian Mayer, Rebecca Gasior Altman, Crystal Adams, Elizabeth Hoover, and Ruth Simpson, "Embodied Health Movements," in *Contested Illnesses: Citizens, Science, and Health Social Movements,* ed. Phil Brown, Rachel Morello-Frosch, and Stephen Zavestoski (Berkeley: University of California Press, 2011), 16.
27. Thomas F. Gieryn, "Boundary-Work and the Demarcation of Science from Non-Science: Strains and Interests in Professional Ideologies of Scientists," *American Sociological Review* 48, no. 6 (1983): 781–95.
28. smith, s. e., "The Beauty of Spaces Created for and by Disabled People," *Catapult,* October 22, 2018, https://magazine.catapult.co.
29. Only one informant identified as nonwhite, although several did not disclose their race at all. It should be noted that seven informants were European citizens, and the racial and gender politics of the United States cannot and should not be cleanly mapped onto these contexts.
30. Siân J. M. Brooke, "Breaking Gender Code: Hackathons, Gender, and the Social Dynamics of Competitive Creation," paper presented at the Association for Computing Machinery's Computer–Human Interaction Conference, 2018, available at https://syllabus.pirate.care/library.
31. Tim Jordan, "A Genealogy of Hacking," *Convergence: The International Journal of Research in New Media Technologies* 23, no. 5 (2016): 1–17.
32. Brooke, "Breaking Gender Code."
33. Steven M. Willi, Kellee M. Miller, Linda A. DiMeglio, Georgeanna J. Klingensmith, Jill H. Simmons, William V. Tamborlane, Kristen J. Nadeau, Julie M. Kittelsrud, Peter Huckfeldt, Roy W. Beck, Terri H. Lipman, and T1D Exchange Clinic Network, "Racial-Ethnic Disparities in Management and Outcomes among Children with Type 1 Diabetes," *Pediatrics* 135, no. 3 (2015): 424–34.
34. Clinical Audit and Registries Management Service, *National Diabetes*

Insulin Audit Report (London: Health and Social Care Information Centre, 2016).

35. Conor Farrington, "Access to Diabetes Technology: The Role of Clinician Attitudes," *Lancet Diabetes Endocrinology* 6, no. 1 (2018): 15.
36. For example, see Andrew Morden, Clare Jinks, and Bie Nio Ong, "Rethinking 'Risk' and Self-Management for Chronic Illness," *Social Theory and Health* 10, no. 1 (2011): 78–99.

CONCLUSION

1. Goodley, *Dis/Ability Studies,* 21–34.
2. Rosemarie Garland-Thomson defines the "normate" as the "corporeal incarnation of the culture's collective, unmarked, normative characteristics." Rosemarie Garland-Thomson, "Integrating Disability, Transforming Feminist Theory," *NWSA Journal* 14, no. 3 (2002): 10.
3. Mateo Pimentel and Rebecca Monteleone, "A Privileged Bodymind: The Entanglement of Ableism and Capitalism," *International Journal of Economic Development* 12, no. 1 (2018): 71.
4. Alison Kafer, "Crip Kin, Manifesting," *Catalyst: Feminism, Theory, Technoscience* 5, no. 1 (2019): 4, https://catalystjournal.org.
5. Inga Bostad and Halvor Hanisch, "Freedom and Disability Rights," *Metaphilosophy* 47, no. 3 (2016): 383.
6. For more on collective liberation through the politicization of disability, see Sins Invalid, *Skin, Tooth, and Bone: The Basis of Movement Is Our People,* 2nd ed. (Berkeley, Calif.: Sins Invalid, 2019).
7. Kafer, *Feminist, Queer, Crip,* 9.
8. Peta Cox, "Passing as Sane, or How to Get People to Sit Next to You on the Bus," in *Disability and Passing: Blurring the Lines of Identity,* ed. Jeffery A. Brune and Daniel J. Wilson (Philadelphia: Temple University Press, 2013), 100, 106.
9. Arseli Dokumacı, *Activist Affordances: How Disabled People Improvise More Habitable Worlds* (Durham, N.C.: Duke University Press, 2023), 250.
10. Kafer, *Feminist, Queer, Crip,* 89.
11. Bowker and Star, *Sorting Things Out.*
12. Conrad, "Medicalization and Social Control."
13. Wendell, *Rejected Body,* 117–38.
14. Annabel Farnood, Bridget Johnston, and Frances S. Mair, "A Mixed Methods Systematic Review of the Effects of Patient Online Self-Diagnosing in the 'Smart-Phone Society' on the Healthcare Professional–Patient Relationship and Medical Authority," *BMC Medical Informatics and Decision Making* 20 (2020), article 253.
15. M. Cameron Hay, R. Jean Cadigan, Dinesh Khanna, Cynthia Strathmann, Eli Lieber, Roy Altman, Maureen McMahon, Morris Kokhab,

and Daniel E. Furst, "Prepared Patients: Internet Information Seeking by New Rheumatology Patients," *Arthritis and Rheumatology* 59, no. 4 (2008): 575–82.

16. Christine Wieseler, "Epistemic Oppression and Ableism in Bioethics," *Hypatia: A Journal of Feminist Philosophy* 35, no. 4 (2004): 714–32.
17. Steven Epstein, "The Construction of Lay Expertise: AIDS Activism and the Forging of Credibility in the Reform of Clinical Trials," *Science, Technology, & Human Values* 20, no. 4 (1995): 408–37.
18. Kristi L. Kirschner and Raymond H. Curry, "Educating Health Care Professionals to Care for Patients with Disabilities," *JAMA* 302, no. 12 (2009): 1334–35.
19. Lisa I. Iezzoni and Linda M. Long-Bellil, "Training Physicians about Caring for Persons with Disabilities: 'Nothing about Us without Us!,'" *Disability and Health Journal* 5, no. 3 (2012): 139.
20. For an example of how disabled people might be included in standardized patient training, see Paula M. Minihan, Ylisabyth S. Bradshaw, Linda M. Long, Wayne Altman, Sonya Perduta-Fulginiti, Jeanette Ector, Karen L. Foran, Lillian Johnson, Paul Kahn, and Robert Sneirson, "Teaching about Disability: Involving Patients with Disabilities as Medical Educators," *Disability Studies Quarterly* 24, no. 1 (2004), https://dsq-sds.org.
21. Goodley, *Dis/Ability Studies,* 160.
22. Shyman, "Reinforcement of Ableism," 368.
23. Heidi L. Janz, "Ableism: The Undiagnosed Malady Afflicting Medicine," *Canadian Medical Association Journal* 191, no. 17 (2019): E478–E479.
24. Gardner and Warren, "Learning from Deep Brain Stimulation," 367.
25. Mia Mingus, "Forced Intimacy: An Ableist Norm," *Leaving Evidence* (blog), August 6, 2017, https://leavingevidence.wordpress.com.
26. Ruth Hubbard, "Abortion and Disability: Who Should and Should Not Inhabit the World?," in Davis, *Disability Studies Reader,* 3rd ed., 107–19.
27. Saxton, "Disability Rights and Selective Abortion," 93.
28. Richard L. Street Jr. and Paul Haidet, "How Well Do Doctors Know Their Patients? Factors Affecting Physician Understanding of Patients' Health Beliefs," *Journal of General Internal Medicine* 26, no. 1 (2011): 21–27.
29. Murphy, *Seizing the Means of Reproduction,* 95–96.
30. Michelle Murphy, "Immodest Witnessing: The Epistemology of Vaginal Self-Examination in the U.S. Feminist Self-Help Movement," *Feminist Studies* 30, no. 1 (2004): 115–47.
31. Gabi Schaffzin, "Reclaiming the Margins in the Face of the Quantified Self," *Review of Disability Studies* 14, no. 2 (2018), https://rdsjournal.org.
32. Mallory Kay Nelson, Ashley Shew, and Bethany Stevens, "Transmo-

bility: Possibilities in Cyborg (Cripborg) Bodies," *Catalyst: Feminism, Theory, Technoscience* 5, no. 1 (2019): 4, https://catalystjournal.org.

33. Stephen Horrocks, "Materializing Datified Body Doubles: Insulin Pumps, Blood Glucose, Testing, and the Production of Usable Bodies," *Catalyst: Feminism, Theory, Technoscience* 5, no. 1 (2019): 5, https://catalystjournal.org.
34. Hamraie and Fritsch, "Crip Technoscience Manifesto," 17.
35. Yergeau, "Disability Hacktivism," para. 24.
36. Gupta, *Medical Entanglements,* 3.
37. Murphy, *Seizing the Means of Reproduction,* 118.
38. Dokumacı, *Activist Affordances,* 245.
39. Dokumacı, *Activist Affordances,* 247.
40. Gupta, *Medical Entanglements,* 4.
41. Goodley, *Dis/Ability Studies,* 169.
42. Hall, *Bioethics of Enhancement,* 139.
43. Margrit Shildrick, *Visceral Prostheses: Somatics and Posthuman Embodiment* (London: Bloomsbury, 2022), 39.

Index

Rebecca Monteleone is associate professor of disability and technology in the Disability Studies Program at the University of Toledo. She is coeditor of *Disability and Social Justice in Kenya: Scholars, Policymakers, and Activists in Conversation*.